Osteoporosis

Harbinger of Chronic Disease

By Dr. David Miller

Dr. David Miller graduated with a B.S. in biology from the Pennsylvania State University. He graduated magna cum laude with a Doctor of Chiropractic degree from New York Chiropractic College and has been in private practice since 1998. He has gained a great appreciation for the importance of addressing problems both metabolically and neurologically in patients, especially those with chronic conditions.

Intended Use Statement

The content of this book is intended for information purposes only. The medical information in this book is intended as general information only and should not be used in any way to diagnose, treat, cure, or prevent any disease. The goal of this book is to present nutritionally significant information and offer suggestions for nutritional support and health maintenance.

It is the sole responsibility of the user of this information to comply with all local and federal laws regarding the use of such information.

Dedication:

To my wonderful wife Maggie for putting up with everything that goes into making dreams come true and to my five precious children - may they bring as much joy to their children.

Contents/ Chapters

"The Doctor of the Future Will Give No Medicine, But Will Interest His Patients in the Care of the Human Frame, In Diet, And in the Cause and Prevention of Disease."

Thomas Edison

Introduction

Our country is sick and our citizens need help. Our current healthcare paradigm is headed for disaster regardless of the political rhetoric tossed about regarding 'healthcare reform'. The problem is we are not really talking about 'healthcare' but 'disease care', and until we differentiate between the two we are headed down the same road to eventually overwhelming our medical resources. We spent over $2.26 trillion in 2007 (and is estimated to be $4.1 trillion by 2016) on sickness care but relatively little on preventative care (about 2 cents out of every healthcare dollar spent). In addition, nearly one third of 'health care' spending is administrative costs. Every measure of health outcomes including longevity, infant mortality, fitness, and rates of chronic diseases puts America at or near the bottom compared to other developed countries. The World Health Organization rated the U.S. 37th in health outcomes, on par with Serbia. The cost of medical care has become a leading cause of bankruptcy; this happens about once every thirty seconds. The Congressional Budget Office reports that 50% of recent increases in the cost of 'health care' are attributable to the introduction of new technology, yet our outcomes remain poor.

We cannot depend on the government for help. These are the same people that brought you the food pyramid, which has been a complete disaster. What evidence is there that 9 - 11 servings of grains a day is healthy?

The FDA has been completely corrupted by pharmaceutical industry interests. Every year the FDA receives 400 million dollars directly from the pharmaceutical industry, thus funding the majority of its budget to review new drugs. The money comes in the form of so-called "user fees" which are payments made by drug companies to encourage the quick review of their drugs. The problem is according to the *Journal of the American Medical Association,* one in five new drugs is found to have significant safety problems *after* it has been approved. This is quite unnerving when you find out that the *average* number of prescriptions per person in 2004 was **twelve.** An FDA official has stated to the non-profit watchdog group Public Citizen, "Everything is approvable. We can use the labeling creatively to lower the problems." Are you kidding? Worse yet, a massive amount of money is spent on direct to consumer (DTC) advertising. In 1995, $595 million was spent on these ads and by 2005 the amount was $3 *billion.* Most of these ads make drugs appear safer and more effective than they actually are. By the way, the U.S. is the only country in the world to allow this kind of advertising. Drug ads are everywhere. In 2000, more was spent on advertising Vioxx® than both Pepsi® and Budweiser®. The FDA didn't seem to want to notice that Vioxx® had caused tens of thousands of serious cardiovascular events, such as heart attacks, and finally issued a warning on August 25, 2004. Eventually, Merck voluntarily pulled Vioxx® from the shelves. The most disturbing part of this is how the FDA approaches medication safety for children. In most cases, Congress lets drug companies decide for themselves whether or not to conduct pediatric studies. Even worse, when the FDA requests that a pharmaceutical company study its drugs to ensure there are no negative side effects on children, those requests are ignored 19% of the time. Bottom line: Nearly two thirds of drugs prescribed for children have not been studied and labeled for pediatric use. (This information comes from the watchdog group Public Citizen - their newsletter Best Pills Worst Pills is a bargain to learn potential problems with medications).

Medicare, the government run health insurance program for the disabled and elderly, is going bankrupt. With all its overwhelming regulation and rules, not to mention its low reimbursement rates, Medicare is putting a tremendous strain on doctors and hospitals. I think it's safe to say that you cannot rely on government to look out for your health.

You also cannot look to insurance companies for true 'healthcare'. An insurance company exists to provide coverage for crisis management and to make money for their shareholders. This is a very expensive approach as it is purely reactive. We can see this with the ever climbing health insurance premiums (along with deductibles and co-payments) at about 20% per year. This is crippling business and our economy. The true responsibility for your health lies in only one place. The true responsibility for your health lies with YOU.

This is why my practice has evolved essentially into a cash practice. I found that I could not adequately diagnose and treat appropriately for the conditions that people were consulting me for under the current insurance model. There is an art component to the practice of healthcare which is being lost and this is what is frustrating many people about our system. One of the biggest complaints I hear from patients that have been to other practitioners is 'Nobody listened to me'. The other big problem is that most doctors don't have enough information from testing to diagnose correctly. Insurance panels do not want 'unnecessary' tests run so doctors order fewer and fewer tests. The American College of Physicians echoes these sentiments in a 2006 report they published: "Medicare payment policies discourage primary care physicians from organizing care processes to achieve optimal results for patients because they are paid little or nothing for the work performed outside of the visit or procedure code; low fees for [evaluation and management] services discourage spending time with patients; prevention is under-reimbursed or not covered at all; low reimbursement coupled with high practice overhead makes it impossible for many primary-care physicians to invest in health-information technology and other practice innovations..." (American College of Physicians, "The Impending Collapse of Primary Care Medicine and Its Implications for the State of the

Nation's Health Care: A Report from the American College of Physicians January 30, 2006). Codes by which Medicare reimburses doctors are used by other insurers and serve as a model for their reimbursement practices. In other words, everyone is using a broken system as their standard which they use to model their procedures on. Does this make any sense? Combine this with the time crunch from managed care (less than five minutes per patient) and you have the perfect storm for failure of the 'healthcare system'.

Doctors are also increasingly frustrated with the system. A recent survey of U.S. primary care physicians found that nearly 50% said they would seriously consider getting out of medicine if they had an alternative.

The main reason why I wrote this book was to give people an alternative way of addressing serious health issues using functional medicine. I try to identify the underlying foundational metabolic issues and give patients a nutritional, neurologic and lifestyle approach to osteoporosis and other chronic conditions. After practicing almost 15 years, this seems to me the only logical way of treating patients. 'An ounce of prevention is worth a pound of cure' is not just a cliché but a truth we need to pay attention to.

Most of the medical community is not on board with this approach, but it should not come as a surprise. It all begins with the way doctors are taught. Nutrition, the pillar of human health, is rarely taught in medical and osteopathic schools. In 2004, *Today's Dietician* performed a survey assessing nutritional education in medical schools. Findings included:

- Only approximately 40% of all osteopathic and medical schools provide a separate, required course in nutrition.
- At schools that require the study of nutrition, the mean number of credit hours was 2.5, with a range of 1 to 10 credits.
- Only 13% of schools offer nutrition as an elective course.
- Nutrition is integrated into other courses at 24% of the colleges.
- Elective courses of 2 credit hours attract less than 25% of the medical school enrollment.
- About 23% of schools do not offer nutrition instruction at all.

[L. Soliah, "A Survey of Nutrition in Medical School Curricula," *Today's Dietitian* 6(2), www.todaysdietition.com/archives/td_204p.20.shtml]

Pharmaceutical companies, on the other hand have a great deal of influence in medical education. They also play a huge role in sponsoring and supporting continuing medical education credits (or CME which each profession is required to take). By 2003, drug companies were spending more than $1500 per year on CME for every doctor in the United States, funding 70% of all continuing education for doctors. It is no wonder doctors have so little information to offer concerning nutrition and exercise/lifestyle management other than 'take calcium and vitamin D' for osteoporosis. This is only one small piece of the puzzle. [For a great book written by an M.D. read *Overdosed America: The Broken Promise of American Medicine* by John Abramson, M.D., Harpercollins 2004]

Another excellent book on the failure of our medical system is Shannon Brownlee's *Overtreated: Why Too Much Medicine Is Making Us Poorer and Sicker* (Bloomsbury 2007). In the book Ms. Brownlee states that the drug industry spends about $25 billion marketing to doctors with one drug rep for every nine doctors with about a $15,000/month expense budget. She goes on to say that one third of academic clinicians have financial ties to either the drug or device industry. Today, the pharmaceutical industry underwrites at least 80% of the clinical research performed. Richard Horton, editor of the prestigious medical journal *Lancet* has stated "Journals have devolved into information laundering operations for the pharmaceutical industry."

David Eddy, a heart surgeon turned mathematician turned healthcare economist and a leader in the evidence-based medicine movement, estimates that as little as 15% of what doctors do is backed by valid evidence.

This is not a book about bashing drug companies, M.D.s, the government or any other group. Thank goodness we do have drugs that when used appropriately can save lives and hospitals to deal with life-threatening situations. We *do* have the best medical trauma system in the world. I am merely saying that *we are overlooking the most important factors in dealing with overwhelming health problems.* Nutrition and lifestyle modification is not fast and sexy but leads to lasting benefits if the patient *works at it!*

I am not a professional writer. When you read this book (warts and all) please remember that this is an effort of one doctor to think outside the box, so to speak, and is a collection of information I have gained from great teachers, colleagues and a lot of reading. If you wish to approach osteoporosis from a different perspective then fasten your seatbelts - you will be in for a wild ride!

Chapter 1

How Bad Is This Problem Really? What's The Big Deal?

Osteoporosis is flying under the radar. It is usually not thought of as life threatening so does not capture a patient's attention unless it leads to a catastrophic event such as a hip fracture. It is also thought of as a disease of the elderly. This is a huge mistake. According to a 400 page report issued by the U.S. Surgeon General, by 2020, "half of all American citizens older than 50 will be at risk for fractures from osteoporosis and low bone mass if no immediate action is taken by individuals at risk, doctors, health systems and policymakers." According to the analysis, an alarming 10 million older Americans suffer from osteoporosis. An additional 34 million are at a high risk of developing the disorder. The report estimates that by 2020, 14 million elderly Americans will have the condition, with an additional 47 million people at high risk. [*U.S. Surgeon General* - October 25, 2004]

Osteoporosis is a disaster which is unfolding now. It is taxing our health care system $17 billion dollars per year and is poised in the next couple of decades to bankrupt our entire medical system if we do not change our paradigm. It is estimated that the cost of osteoporosis treatment will increase to more than $100 billion by the year 2040. We hear about drug treatments, calcium supplements and some of the consequences of bone loss, but do we really care?

The National Women's Health Resource Center (NWHRC) released a survey that found while women view osteoporosis as a serious and preventable health threat, few women clearly understand the effects and causes of bone loss. Even though the majority of women in the survey said they exercise and take calcium to prevent bone loss, few seemed to understand or fear the consequences of not having healthy bones. "Now that we are aware of the causes and dangers inherent in osteoporosis, millions of women will continue to disregard vital research studies, which point to the negative effects of the disease without intervention," says John Amarco, D.C., FIAMA. "It is our duty as DCs to educate our female patients to the seriousness of bone loss and guide them in prevention and treatment." The national survey found that women are waiting until it is too late to make a connection between bone loss and spinal fractures. Also according to the survey, women believe they are not at risk for spinal fracture when, in fact, a Caucasian woman over the age of 50 has a 40% chance of suffering a fracture at some point in her life. I would contend that men are completely oblivious to this disease.

How is medicine doing with prevention? An article from the *Tufts University Health and Nutrition Letter* October 2003 gives us some insight. The article asks: Has your physician ever asked you whether your mother or sister suffered a bone fracture as a result of fragility? Have you been counseled on calcium or nutrition? Have you been asked if you are doing the appropriate amount of exercise for bone strengthening? There's probably a good chance that this is not happening. Even women who have already suffered a fracture (raising the risk of a second fracture four to seven fold within the first year) are often not adequately advised or treated says Dr. Bess Dawson-Hughes, M.D., president of the National Osteoporosis Foundation and chief of the Bone Metabolism Laboratory at Tuft's USDA Human Nutrition Research Center on Aging. Consider one study in which only 7% to 37% of patients at four different hospitals were put on medication within a year of suffering a hip fracture, even though prescriptions in such cases are supposed to be standard treatment. (Whether the drugs work or not is another story which we will discuss later). In another study, only 27% of women with hip fractures were given appropriate medical treatment. The statistics "have run from horrible to dismal," Dr. Dawson-Hughes states.

Let's look at screening. An article from *Tufts University Health and Nutrition Letter* May 2008 stated that women who could most benefit from osteoporosis screening are the least likely to get it, according to the study cited. Researchers at the Medical College of Wisconsin in Milwaukee found that as women age they are less likely to be screened for the bone thinning condition. In an analysis of 44,000 women, the investigators found that 27% of those age 66 to 70 were screened in a three year period. Less than 10% of the oldest women, ages 80 to 90, were screened. The risk of osteoporosis jumps with age, afflicting less than 20% of women 65 to 74 but more than 50% of women over the age of 85. According to the lead author Joan M. Neuner, M.D., MPH, 40% of Caucasian women age 50 and older will suffer an osteoporosis related fracture of the hip, wrist or spine at some point in their lifetime. More than half of those with hip fractures never fully recover, and 20% will end up in a nursing home. So most don't care about the disease, we don't screen for it, doctors don't talk about. Yet, osteoporosis is poised to bankrupt our entire medical system in the near future if we do not change course. Interesting.

Another point to consider. Osteoporosis does not show up overnight. It is preceded by a precursor 'condition' called osteopenia. This is like metabolic syndrome is to diabetes. This adds many more people to the potential osteoporosis patient pool. On September 28, 2003, Gina Kolata, a science writer for the *New York Times*, outlined several points concerning osteopenia in her article:

- The disease, if it is a disease, afflicts mostly middle - aged and elderly women, and a large segment of men. But it has no symptoms, and it is not clear what patients should do about it and it is being diagnosed more and more often.
- The condition is osteopenia, or low bone density. It is considered by many doctors to be a first step along the path to osteoporosis, a serious condition in which bone density is extremely low and bones are porous and prone to shatter. But researchers say that while bone density predicts fracture risk, <u>more is involved,</u> including age, family history and a poorly understood factor known as **bone quality**.
- The stakes are particularly high with osteopenia because the number of patients is enormous. One

federal study in which more than 14,000 men and women were screened estimated, conservatively, that osteopenia afflicts 13 million to 17 million women and 1 million to 2 million men in this country.

- Also at stake is the calcium supplement market. Many people take calcium supplements in the hope of staving off bone loss. Researchers say that calcium may have a small effect but is not going to obliterate the effects of menopause or aging. (We will discuss this later)

For all intents and purposes, osteoporosis is a silent thief only becoming evident when a catastrophic event, like a fracture, occurs. However, a woman's risk of developing an osteoporosis related injury is equal to her *combined* risk of developing breast, ovarian or uterine cancer.

Consequences of Decreased Bone Mass

✓ Responsible for 1.3 million fractures per year in patients over the age of 45

✓ Risk of embolism

✓ By extreme old age, one of every three women and one of every six men will have had a hip fracture which, by any measure, is the most devastating of all osteoporotic fractures

✓ Osteoporosis is responsible for 300,000 hip fractures, 700,000 vertebral fractures, and 250,000 wrist fractures per year

✓ Of the 300,000 hip fractures, 50% of those individuals will never walk without assistance again, up to 30%

will be unable to live independently, and another 25% will die within one year
✓ The incidence of hip fractures in women doubles every five years after the age of 60

The bottom line is osteoporosis is a serious and devastating condition which is going unchecked. It is important to remember that osteoporosis is almost always due to some other condition; it is usually not the primary problem. In functional medicine we must uncover the underlying causes which may be leading to osteoporosis, not merely to tell the patient to take calcium and exercise.

Chapter 2

Why Do People Get Osteoporosis?

In this chapter we will discuss why people get osteoporosis and the complex physiology behind some of the reasons that may not be initially clear.

Factors For Increased Risk Of Osteoporosis

- ✓ Female
- ✓ Menopausal
- ✓ Small frame
- ✓ Oophorectomy, or menopause by age 45
- ✓ Prolonged hormonal imbalances
- ✓ Known calcium, mineral and vitamin D deficiencies
- ✓ Insufficient physical activity
- ✓ Caucasian or Asian ancestry - genetics (strong family history)
- ✓ Smoker
- ✓ Excess caffeine intake (more than 3 cups of coffee, tea or soda/day)
- ✓ More than 2 alcoholic drinks per day
- ✓ Regular use of certain medications (glucocorticoids, thyroid hormone, anticonvulsants and aluminum containing antacids)
- ✓ History of eating disorders
- ✓ Nulliparous women (no children)
- ✓ Dental problems (soft teeth, receding gums, periodontal disease, shattering teeth, tooth plaque, eroding jawbone, etc.)

- ✓ Barbituate use
- ✓ Chronic renal failure
- ✓ Chronic obstructive pulmonary disease
- ✓ Rheumatoid arthritis
- ✓ Malignancy and certain chemotherapy medications
- ✓ Hyperparathyroidism
- ✓ Diabetes mellitus
- ✓ Heparin use
- ✓ Malabsorption syndrome and Celiac disease/gluten reactivity)
- ✓ Sarcoidosis
- ✓ Testosterone deficiency (in men)

What determines bone density? It is a combination of genetics and environment/lifestyle. We cannot blame everything on genes. Genetics can account for 60 - 80% of our bone density, which means that up to 40% of our bone density is determined by lifestyle choices. Genetics can affect bone density in the following way. About 19% of people have a variant of a gene named CYP1A1 that appears to boost the risk of osteoporosis. (*Journal of Bone and Mineral Research* February 2005; 20: 232-239) In women, the variant hastens the breakdown of estrogen and is associated with low density of the hip. "Previous studies showed that some CYP1A1 variants are linked to estrogen related cancers, such as breast, ovarian or endometrial cancers," says primary researcher Reina Armamento - Villareal, M.D. "The link to estrogen suggested that the gene could also affect bone density." Think of it as genetics loading the gun but environment lifestyle pulling the trigger.

It turns out, however, that the most important factor for bone health is lifestyle. A study in the *Journal of Epidemiology and Community Health* revealed the critical factor seems to be adult lifestyle. (*Journal of Epidemiology and Community Health* June 2005; 59: 475 - 480) No matter how much we want to look for the magic bullet it comes down to education and work.

We cannot discount how important the childhood years are in bone health. This is why osteoporosis is really a young person's condition. The choices you make in childhood and adolescence will dictate your future bone mass and bone health. Peak growth occurs at age 12 - 16 in boys and 11 - 13 in girls. 45% of a young person's skeletal mass is formed during this period of adolescence. By age 20, 98% of a woman's skeletal mass is established. This is also the time of some of the worst nutritional habits with deficiencies being epidemic, especially nutrients such as calcium and iron. One in three kids eat fast food every day and 19% of American meals are eaten in a car.

The first risk factor that is completely under our control and one of the most important when speaking of health in general is smoking. This should not come as a shock. How does smoking influence bone health? A 1982 article in the *New England Journal of Medicine* discovered the levels of three major estrogens were reduced during the second half of the menstrual cycle in women who smoked. Another study in 1986 found evidence that women who smoked could not make estrogen in the ovaries with the same efficiency as nonsmokers. In premenopausal women smoking may:

- Decrease the production of estrogen in the ovaries
- Cause estrogen to be changed chemically in the liver rendering it useless
- Cause an earlier menopause and total cessation of estrogen production in the ovaries (2 years earlier)

This factor absolutely must be addressed from the beginning. I will not accept a patient for nutritional work if they smoke since health and smoking are incompatible.

Where It All Begins - Children

Let's be clear. You cannot have bad habits during childhood and end up as a healthy adult. There are certain windows of opportunity during these years (like building peak bone mass and decreasing the risk of obesity) which we may not be able to make up for in adulthood. These periods are gestation and early infancy, the period of 5 to 7 years of age, and adolescence. Problems like obesity that begin at these periods tend to be persistent. (*Experimental Physiology* 2007, 92(2): 287-298, *American Journal of Clinical Nutrition* 1994 May; 59(5): 955-9, *Proceedings of the National Academy of Sciences* 2006; 103(17): 6676-6681)   I'm not saying you can't change and correct many heath issues as an adult, but you are starting off at a distinct disadvantage. In this section we will explore some of the issues affecting bone health in children.

I'm sure you have heard of kids having 'growing pains' but you may not be aware that these pains are linked with lower bone density. This comes from the *Journal of Rheumatology* July 2005; 32: 1354-7. Children with 'growing pains' have weaker bones than their peers without this condition. According to the study's authors, recurring childhood musculoskeletal leg pain may be an overuse syndrome, which is provoked by activities such as running and jumping. If growing pains are an overuse syndrome, kids with weaker leg bones would be more susceptible to these aches, speculated the study's authors. To test this hypothesis, they evaluated the bone strength of 39 youngsters with growing pains. Results revealed that 28% of children with growing pains had below average bone density. Bone density was particularly low in spots on the shin where children reported the pain. Although exercise may incite growing pains, it should not be avoided because it will strengthen the leg bones and reduce the risk of overuse pain, stress the study's authors.

One of the biggest components to bone health in children is physical activity. Children who engage in high impact exercises, such as running, grow to have stronger bones, compared with youngsters who do not participate in high impact activities. In addition, the bone strengthening benefits of early exercises persist even when exercise is discontinued later in life. [*Journal of Bone and Mineral Research* November 13, 2006]

A growing trend related to many factors such as computers, TV, video games has led to decreased activity. Look at the following statistics:

- Nearly half of young people ages 12 - 21, and more than one third of high school students, do not participate in vigorous physical activity on a regular basis.
- Fewer than one in four children get 20 minutes of physical activity every day, and report at least half an hour of any type of physical activity every day of the week.
- One out of four children do not attend any school physical education classes and only one in three get physical activity every day.
- Fourteen percent of children ages 6 - 11 are overweight, while 12% of adolescents ages 12 - 17 are overweight.
- The percentage of overweight young Americans has more than doubled in the past 30 years.
- After smoking, physical inactivity is the single largest health risk factor in the country today.
- Obesity related diseases cost the United States economy more than $100 billion per year.

Other, less obvious factors may come in to play such as surgeries like tonsillectomies. Children who undergo tonsillectomies are significantly more likely to become overweight, compared with children who do not have their tonsils removed, according to a report in the journal

Pediatrics (April 2009; 123: 1095-1101). Tonsillectomy with or without adenoidectomy boosted a child's odds of being overweight at age 8 by 61%, and of being obese by 136%. Adenoidectomy without tonsillectomy did not increase the likelihood of being overweight, but did increase the odds of developing obesity by 94%.

These factors can be changed to have a positive impact. An article in the journal *International Journal of Sports Medicine 2006; 27, 666 - 671* examined how a combination of dietary and physical activity interventions affect bone strength in obese children and adolescents. Other studies have shown obese children and adolescents are at risk for decreased bone strength and bone mineral density (BMD). Researchers in this study examined the effects of a combined nutritional/physical activity intervention on bone strength in obese children and adolescents. All subjects participated in assessments prior to and upon completion of the three month intervention. Assessments consisted of body mass index (BMI), percent fat, dietary intake (2 day food record), exercise endurance (progressive treadmill test), and bone strength determined using quantitative ultrasound measurements of bone speed of sound (SOS). The intervention group had a significant increase in bone SOS vs. the control group which actually had a significant decrease in bone SOS. This study demonstrates that a short term nutrition and physical activity program for obese children and adolescents can bring about significant desired changes in weight, BMI, body fat, fitness and bone strength. These results emphasize the importance of physical activity and dietary intervention for the treatment of childhood obesity and its complications.

How does obesity harm bones? Dr. Hong-Wen Deng of the University of Missouri in Kansas City, and colleagues from China, showed that obesity can accelerate bone loss. The finding undermines prior assumptions that obesity made skeletons stronger and more resistant to fractures. Deng's research showed that the bone strengthening benefits of a heavy body aren't due to fat, as some might have assumed, but to elevated muscle mass, which increases bone density. Higher fat content was linked to weaker bones, which are more prone to fractures. (This makes sense if you think about it. In order to achieve greater muscle mass there would have to be some type of resistance training to stimulate muscle growth thereby creating force on a bone and therefore growing stronger by Wolff's Law. Wolff's Law states: A bone, normal or abnormal, develops the structure most suited to resist the forces acting upon it. You can increase body fat without physical training thereby increasing weight but minimizing physical stress on the bones.)

In the last 50 years the trend of increasing obesity has been astounding. Go to the CDC's website and look at how fast each state in the country has increased its obesity rate. (www.cdc.gov) The fastest growing segment of America's overweight population is also the fattest. A Rand Corporation study reports that the biggest growth area among people that are overweight is the group that's extremely obese, 100 or more pounds too heavy. The report, which is published in the journal *Public Health,* says the population of Americans with a body mass index (BMI) of 50 or more increased by 75% between 2000 and 2005. Rand researcher Roland Sturm noted, "The proportion of people at the high end of the weight scale continues to increase at a brisk rate despite increased public attention on the risks of obesity and the increased use of drastic weight loss strategies such as bariatric surgeries." The number of bariatric procedures, including stomach stapling and stomach bypass surgery, rose from 13,000 in 1998 to an estimated 200,000 last year, the report notes [*Tufts University Health and Nutrition Letter* June 2007]

Patients need to be careful regarding dieting and calorie restriction, however. Individuals at potential risk of spinal bone quality problems who want to lose weight might do well to opt for weight loss through exercise rather than dieting. Dennis T. Villareal, M.D., et al. randomly allocated 48 moderately overweight middle - aged adults to one of three interventions: (1) weight loss through calorie restriction; (2) weight loss through regular exercise; and (3) a healthy lifestyle control group. At the end of a year, subjects who cut calories lost an average of 18.1 pounds and those who exercised lost 14 pounds while the healthy lifestyle group maintained baseline weight levels. However, the weight loss in the calorie restriction group came at a cost. Individuals in this group lost an average of 2.2% of their bone density in the lumbar spine, 2.2% at the hip, and 2.1% at the top of the femur. Neither the exercise group nor the healthy lifestyle group showed any changes in bone density. (See *Archives of*

Internal Medicine, 2006; 166: 2502-10) Previous studies have suggested that dieting may promote bone loss through the reduction of mechanical stress on the weight bearing skeleton. (Remember Wolff's Law?) The exercise group managed to avoid this effect, at least in this study. The loading imposed by exercise may strengthen the bones enough that it counterbalances the loss of skeletal loading imposed by a decrease in body weight. [*The Back Letter* Vol. 22, No. 1 January 2007]

Another epidemic looming which has a huge impact on osteoporosis is that of diabetes and metabolic syndrome. The increase in the prevalence of type 2 diabetes is closely linked to the upsurge in obesity. About 90% of type 2 diabetes is attributable to excess weight. Furthermore, approximately 197 million people worldwide have impaired glucose tolerance, most commonly because of obesity and the associated metabolic syndrome. This number is expected to increase to 420 million by 2025. Diabetes is rapidly emerging as a global health care problem that threatens to reach pandemic levels by 2030. The number of people with diabetes worldwide is projected to increase from 171 million in 2000 to 366 million by 2030. In the U.S. and Canada, there were 19.7 million diabetics in 2000 and this is projected to increase to 33.9 million in 2030. For every Caucasian child born in the U.S. in 2000, one third will be diabetic. For African Americans and Latinos, that statistic climbs to one half of children born in 2000. [*New England Journal of Medicine* 356;3 January 18, 2007] Treatment of diabetes can be a risk for osteoporosis according to the FDA. Women who are prescribed Avandia® should take note: The drug poses dangers to their health in addition to the well publicized risks of heart failure or heart attacks and also increases the chances of a bone fracture. The FDA issued warnings about the increased risk of upper arm, hand and foot fractures in women who use the type 2 diabetes drug Avandia® (rosiglitazone) or the related diabetes drug Actos® (pioglitazone).

It doesn't get better for college aged women either. These early habits have a lasting effect in addition to eating disorders and birth control issues. Research from the University of Arkansas Fayetteville (July 31, 2002) revealed that 2% of college age women already have osteoporosis. A further 15% have osteopenia, setting them up for osteoporosis. At highest risk of low bone density were women who maintained low body mass index through dieting and who did not exercise. The study also found that Depo-Provera, a common method of birth control that consists of hormone injections every three months, was associated with significant bone loss, especially with long term use.

Men are certainly not immune to this problem. Osteoporosis commonly seen as a woman's illness yet, is a very common problem in men. How common? One in every eight men above the age of 50 will suffer a hip fracture as a result of osteoporosis. Part of the problem is a lack of screening and subsequent treatment; the number of men screened at bone mineral density labs is quite few. Men's osteoporosis is often the outcome of another illness, especially one that requires treatment with drugs like corticosteroids or anticonvulsants. Both are notorious for thinning bone. Also at high risk are tobacco users and heavy drinkers. The two habits, linked with fractures from the disease, are more common in men than in women. [*Tufts University Health and Nutrition Letter* August 2003]

Men also have to contend with prostate cancer. In an article published in the *Journal of Clinical Endocrinology and Metabolism* June 2001:87, the authors were surprised to find that men who were treated with GnRH-a for prostate cancer experienced up to a decade's worth of bone loss within the first year of therapy. In treating men with this therapy earlier and for longer periods of time, we are putting them in a menopause equivalent condition and subjecting them to severe osteoporosis - a disease that may have more serious consequences than early stage prostate cancer. With close to 200,000 men being diagnosed with prostate cancer each year, we could be facing an enormous increase in the incidence of debilitating bone fractures in men.

Another area where fracture risk is greatly elevated is the treatment of depression. Prescription drugs often have side effects that seem completely unrelated to their function. This is because they affect the entire body, not just the part that's being treated. Examples are antacids causing pneumonia and osteoporosis, eye drops causing heart arrhythmias, COX-2 anti-inflammatories causing heart attacks, thalidomide causing birth deformities, and now depression drugs causing fractures in older adults. We have long known about this side effect, but a study in the *Archives of Internal Medicine* (January 22, 2007) brings it back into focus. It showed that drugs like Zoloft®, Prozac®, and others **doubled the risk** of broken bones. And researchers did their best to eliminate other fracture risks in the study participants. Antidepressants have been linked with low blood pressure and dizziness, which can obviously cause falls and broken bones. But the fracture risk in this study was independent of these factors. For years medical researchers have felt that these pills actually have a direct effect on bone cells themselves - making them smaller and weaker. Since millions of Americans are prescribed antidepressants annually, and in steadily increasing numbers, these results have major public health implications. Indeed, severe depression is serious and while drugs are rarely the long term solution, they are often necessary, even if temporary. This is one of the reasons good nutrition is essential. [*Health Alert* - Dr. Bruce West April 2007 Vol. 24, Issue 4]

An additional study to reinforce this idea found that drugs used to treat depression and other mental illnesses may heighten the risk of fractures. Dr. Brent Richards from McGill University, working with researchers in the Canadian Multicentre Osteoporosis Study presented the findings. According to the study's results, daily use of selective serotonin reuptake inhibitors (SSRIs) - which rank among the most widely prescribed drugs in the world with combined annual sales of $8.3 billion - were associated with an elevated risk of x-ray confirmed fragility fractures among subjects aged 50 years and above. "The take home message is that SSRI use, depression and fractures are common in the elderly," Richards says. "So, given these high prevalences, the risk of fractures may have important public health implications."

A significant number of people will have hip fractures due to medications for gastro-esophageal reflux disease (GERD). A study published in the *Journal of the American Medical Association* December 27, 2006; 296: 2947-53 links a widely used medication called an acid suppressing proton pump inhibitor (PPIs) for GERD with a bolstered risk of hip fracture. PPIs are particularly popular among individuals with back and other forms of chronic pain who take these meds in an effort to counteract and/or prevent serious GI complications associated with long term NSAID use. (Note that between 16,000 and 20,000 people die every year from gastrointestinal bleeding from NSAIDS *The New England Journal of Medicine* June 17, 1999 page 1888) Residents of the United States alone filled some 95 million prescriptions for PPIs in 2005, to the tune of roughly $12.8 billion dollars. They also spent another $1.9 million on Prilosec®, a PPI available on an over the counter basis. The findings of the study revealed that the use of proton pump inhibitors increased the likelihood of hip fracture by 44%. The longer the use of the drugs, the greater the risk. The study's authors speculate that the drugs may interfere with calcium metabolism.

This makes sense if you think about the physiology. We need strong stomach acid to break apart or ionize minerals in order to absorb them. Without this acid, people are unable to absorb any significant amount of calcium and other minerals especially if the mineral takes multiple steps to ionize such as calcium carbonate. Calcium lactate, on the other hand, takes only one step to ionize and only needs a weak stomach acid to achieve this. It's not the amount of calcium we take that is important, but the amount we can absorb and utilize. Another issue stemming from decreased stomach acid is the inability to digest protein. When undigested protein reaches the intestines, bacteria produce gas and organic acids which may add to the GERD along with bloating and other GI unpleasantness about one half hour after eating. Stomach acid also has the job of killing bacteria, viruses and other bugs that are normally swallowed with our food. Without this protection our stomach and intestines become more vulnerable to infection by organisms like Helobactor pylori.

Some Less Well Known Reasons For Osteoporosis

Fluoride and Bone Fractures

When fluoride is ingested, approximately 93% of it is absorbed into the bloodstream. A good part of this intake is excreted, but the rest is deposited in the bones and teeth and is capable of causing skeletal fluorosis. Because some symptoms of skeletal fluorosis mimic arthritis, the first two clinical phases of fluorosis can easily be misdiagnosed.

Radiologic changes in bone can occur when fluoride exposure is 5 mg. per day. While 5 mg. per day is the amount of fluoride ingested by living in fluoridated areas, the number increases for diabetics and laborers, who can ingest up to 20 mg. daily.

Three studies reported in the *Journal of the American Medical Association* showed links between hip fractures and fluoride. A 1992 study, for example, found a 'small but significant increase in the risk of hip fractures in both men and women exposed to artificial fluoridation at 1 ppm'. In addition, the *New England Journal of Medicine* has reported that people given fluoride to cure their osteoporosis actually end up with an increased non-vertebral fracture rate. Austrian researchers have also found that fluoride tablets make bones more susceptible to fractures. [*The Townsend Letter* January 2003]

Scientists at Yale University discovered that doses as low as 1 part per million (ppm) of fluoride decrease bone strength and elasticity, making fractures more likely. Two studies published in the early 1990s found that the rate of hip fracture generally increased with exposure to fluoridated water, and the results of more recent studies have suggested that fluoride in water will increase the risk of hip fractures for certain age groups of women. Of eighteen studies conducted since 1990 on the possible link between fluoride and a greater rate of hip fractures in the elderly, ten have found such an association.

Fluoride may increase bone quantity but also decrease bone quality and bone strength. It is well known that pharmacological doses of fluoride increase the risk of torsion type fractures (such as hip fractures) despite the appearance of greater bone density. (This concept will come up again when we discuss the bisphosphonate drugs used for treating osteoporosis) In an experiment on cow bone, fluoride treatment reduced the mechanical strength of bone tissue by converting small amounts of bone mineral to mostly calcium fluoride. This action structurally reduces the effective bone mineral content and possibly affects the interface bonding between the bone mineral and the organic matrix of the bone tissue. When combined with a calcium deficiency, the effect of fluoride may be even worse.

Cadmium and Bone

Cadmium is considered one of the most toxic substances in the environment due to its wide range of organ toxicity and long elimination half-life of 10 to 30 years. Cadmium contaminated topsoil is considered the most likely mechanism for the greatest human exposure through uptake into edible plants and tobacco. Fertilizer raw materials are also contaminated with cadmium along with rubber tire dust and other industrial waste. The uptake of cadmium from soil through produce results in elevated concentrations in vegetables, fruits, and grains with the highest levels in leafy greens and potatoes. Iron deficiency creates a significant risk for increased cadmium exposure by increasing gastrointestinal absorption from 5% to as much as 20%.

The cadmium content of human bone in North America has increased by a factor of 50 in the last 600 years. Classic cadmium poisoning (known as itai-itai disease in Japan) has been characterized by multiple fractures, osteomalacia (thinning bone), bone pain, and osteoporosis that occurs along with renal disease. Epidemiological studies have found a positive correlation with elevated urinary cadmium and increased urinary calcium loss. The mechanisms behind cadmium and bone loss are related to renal tubular cell damage that results in elevated levels of urinary calcium and lowered levels of vitamin D3. Lower levels of activated vitamin D3 alter calcium homeostasis by decreasing absorption of calcium in the gut and altering deposition in bone.

Homocysteine and Fracture Risk

High blood levels of homocysteine have already been linked with cardiovascular disease, cancer and cognitive decline. Now a paper in the *New England Journal of Medicine* ties the amino acid with osteoporosis related bone fracture. After controlling for risk factors of fracture such as body mass index, smoking, age and gender, the scientists calculated that homocysteine significantly ups the odds of fracture. The risk was similar in men and women. 'An increased homocysteine level appears to be a strong and independent risk factor for osteoporotic fractures in older men and women,' concludes the study's authors. [*NEJM* May 15, 2004; 350: 2033-41]

LDL Cholesterol and Bone Density

Postmenopausal women with elevated blood levels of low density lipoprotein (LDL) cholesterol may want to watch out for thinning bones. According to research from the University of Milan, these women may be at increased risk for osteopenia or reduced bone density that precedes osteoporosis. Women with LDL's above 160 were much more likely to be osteopenic than women with normal or low LDL's (below 130). Neither total nor high density lipoprotein (HDL) cholesterol was linked to osteopenia. LDL's may alter bone metabolism so that normal everyday bone breakdown exceeds bone formation, the researchers suggest. These findings could explain why cholesterol - lowering drugs and nutritional support appear to improve bone density. [*Environmental Nutrition* December 2003 Vol. 26 Number 12]

With the hype regarding cholesterol and statin drugs, one thing should be kept in mind. When a statin drug shuts down the enzyme HMG reductase which prevents the liver from making cholesterol, it also cuts the activity of alkaline phosphatase, an enzyme essential for bone osteoblastic activity (bone building activity) almost in half - a clinical disaster. This was published in *Cardiovascular Drugs Ther.* 2009 August 23(4) 295-9 but the detail regarding alkaline phosphatase was not well publicized. I wonder why?

Osteoporosis and Memory

This is not a cause but I wanted to show the interrelatedness of the functions of the body. Researchers calculated that subjects with the highest bone mineral density were 44% less likely to have memory problems, compared to those with the weakest bones. [*American Journal of* Epidemiology November 1, 2001; 154: 795]

Nutritional Reasons for Osteoporosis

Carbonated Beverage Consumption

A study by the Harvard Medical School and the Harvard School of Public Health confirmed previous findings that consumption of cola drinks are associated with bone fractures in physically active girls (mean age of 15 years 8 months). Interestingly, the researchers observed that for less active girls, the associations between carbonated cola beverages and bone fractures is marginal; however, for active girls that consume both cola and non-cola drinks, the risk of bone fractures is the highest. Teens have tripled their consumption of soft drinks and have cut their consumption of milk by more than 40%. These findings have implications for the health of women at later ages. [*Arch Pediatric Adol Medicine* 2000; 154: 610-613]

Colas are not any better for older women either. According to an assessment of 1,413 women and 1,125 men, cola (but not other carbonated beverages) may trigger osteoporosis in older women. In women, cola consumption was associated with lower bone mineral density at all three hip sites tested, regardless of factors such as age, menopausal status, total calcium and vitamin D intake, or uses of cigarettes or alcohol. However, cola consumption was not associated with a lower bone mineral density for men at the hip sites, or the spine for either men or women. The results are similar for diet cola, and, although weaker, for decaffeinated cola as well. "The more cola that women drank, the lower their bone mineral density was," noted study author Katherine Tucker, PhD.

[*American Journal of Clinical Nutrition* October 2006; 84: 936-42]

Osteoporosis and Essential Fatty Acids (Fish Oils)

A review article [*Prog Lipid Res* 1997 Sept.; 36(2-3): 131-51] points out that essential fatty acid (EFA) deficient animals develop severe osteoporosis, coupled with an increased renal and arterial calcification. This is also one of the reasons why EFAs are important in cardiovascular disease. This picture is similar to that seen in the elderly, where loss of bone calcium is associated with calcification of the soft tissues, especially arteries and kidneys. The same review article points out that EFAs have been shown to increase calcium absorption from the gut. They do so in part by enhancing the effects of vitamin D. The article goes on to say that EFAs reduce urinary calcium excretion, increase calcium deposition in bone, improve bone strength and enhance the synthesis of bone collagen. These benefits of EFAs are associated with one other benefit, namely, that there is reduced soft tissue calcification when EFAs are adequately present. (Another good review of research is *Nutrition* 2000 May; 16(5): 386-90)

The problem of essential (meaning we cannot make them - they are required in our diet) fats today is the ratio of omega-6 to omega-3 is much too high. The intake of omega-6 (corn oil, soybean oil, safflower oil, sunflower oil) has doubled in Europe, America, and other affluent populations over the last 100 years due to increased use of these oils in food preparation. On the other hand, omega-3 intake (EPA/DHA from fish oils, flaxseed oil and alpha-linolenic acid) has been reduced to less than 20% of what people ate 150 years ago.

Medium Chain Fatty Acids

Medium chain fatty acids (MCFAs) like those found in coconut oil enhance the absorption of calcium and magnesium as well as amino acids. This is one of the reasons coconut oil is used in baby formulas and in hospitals for patients that have gastric problems. It is also used for those children suffering from rickets which is a bone demineralizing disease caused by a lack of vitamin D.

Researchers from Purdue University found that free radicals from oxidized vegetable oils interfere with bone formation, thus contributing to osteoporosis. They also found that vitamin E protects the bones from free radicals. Medium chain saturated fats (coconut oil) also act as antioxidants to protect the bones. (For more in depth information on coconut oil, read *The Coconut Oil Miracle* by Bruce Fife, C.N., N.D.)

Vitamin K and Bone Strength

A Dutch study suggests that menaquinone-4, a form of vitamin K, may be another tool to help maintain bone strength in postmenopausal women. In a three year study of 325 healthy older women, the researchers found that those taking supplements of menaquinone-4 maintained hip bone strength, while women on a placebo suffered weakening. Vitamin K comes in two main forms: Vitamin K1, phylloquinne, is found in leafy green vegetables and makes up about 90% of our dietary vitamin K. Menaquinone-4 is an example of the second type of vitamin K, a complex of vitamins known as menaquinones, which the body can synthesize naturally. Meat, cheese and the Japanese food natto are among the dietary sources.

Further support for menaquinones come from a double blind study, published in *Osteoporosis International,* compared the effects of a high dose (45 mg.) of supplements of menaquinone-4 against a placebo. In the treated group, "hip bone strength remain unchanged during the three year period, whereas in the placebo group bone strength decreased significantly," the researcher reported. While no benefit was seen for bone mineral density, women in the menaquinone-4 group also showed better compression strength, bending strength, impact strength and femoral neck width than those in the placebo group. Overall, the menaquinone-4 supplements seemed to help women maintain their bone strength even as bone mineral density naturally decreased after menopause. This gives credence to the idea that there is more to bone health than just bone density. It is about bone quality.

Several studies support the link between vitamin K and osteoporosis. A study in *Menopause* (September 2006; 13: 799-808) suggests that not enough vitamin K compromises bone health and contributes to the development of osteoporosis. The study found that one of the early effects of declining estrogen is the impairment of vitamin K function in bone - even before any bone loss can be detected. "Our study suggests that the generally accepted level of vitamin K in healthy women is inadequate to maintain bone health just at the onset of menopause," researcher Jane Lukacs comments. She notes that while most multivitamins do not contain vitamin K, the nutrient may be obtained through green vegetables and vegetable oils.

The Nurses Health Study followed more than 72,000 women for 10 years. Investigators found that women whose vitamin K intake was in the lowest quintile had a 30% higher risk of hip fractures than women with vitamin K intakes in the highest four quartiles. (*Fescanich D., et al. American Journal of Clinical Nutrition* 1999 69(1): 74-79) Another study that showed the relationship between reduced blood plasma vitamin K levels and hip fracture is *Lancet* 2:283, 1984.

Food Sources of Vitamin K

Cheese	Collard greens
Liver	Spinach
Asparagus	Salad greens
Coffee	Kale
Bacon	Broccoli
Green tea	Brussels sprouts
Cabbage	Olive oil
Cauliflower	Okra

Cereals   Green beans

Soybeans   Lentils

*Also made by bacteria in the gut

Magnesium and Osteoporosis

Approximately half of the total magnesium pool in the body is present intracellularly in the soft tissues and the other half is present in the bone. Consistent with animal studies, numerous population studies demonstrate a positive association between magnesium intake and bone mineral density. It has been found that magnesium intake was positively associated with hip bone mineral density in both men and women of the original Framingham Heart Study cohort. Magnesium is involved in over 300 different enzymatic reactions in the body.

Magnesium Content of Food

Food	Magnesium (mg.)
Pumpkin seeds, ¼ cup roasted	303
Almonds, ½ cup	238
Soy nuts, ½ cup	196
Cashews, ½ cup	157

Tofu, firm, ½ cup	128
Peanuts, ½ cup	125
Chili with beans, 1 cup	115
Molasses, 2 tbsp.	100
Wheat germ, toasted, 2 tbsp.	90
Unsweetened chocolate, 1 oz.	88
Sunflower seeds, ¼ cup	82
Halibut, baked, 3 oz.	78
Swiss chard, cooked, ½ cup	75
Spinach, ½ cup cooked	66
Black beans, ½ cup	60
Oatmeal, 1 cup cooked	56
Peanut butter, 2 Tbsp.	51
Baked potato with skin, 1	55
Cereal, raisin bran, 1 oz.	48
Low fat yogurt, 1 cup	43
Milk, nonfat, 1 cup	28
Chicken, breast, 3 oz.	25

Iron and Bone Health

There is another bone strengthening mineral besides calcium worthy of attention: iron. Scientists at the Universities of Arizona and Arkansas along with investigators at Columbia University found that women whose daily iron consumption hovered around 18 mg. had the greatest bone mineral density. (The postmenopausal RDA is 8 mg.) Why would iron be so important for bone mineral density? It promotes the production of collagen, a central component of bone. The finding that iron intake is associated with higher bone density held true for women who consumed between 800 and 1,200 mg. of calcium daily. More or less calcium with that much iron did not appear to be of any bone building help. The most important factor appears to be mineral balance, cites the lead researcher. [*Tufts University Health and Nutrition Newsletter* January 2004, Vol. 21, No. 11]

Phosphorus and Bone Health

Research presented at the National Osteoporosis Foundation's Fifth International Symposium in Hawaii showed for the first time that calcium and phosphorus are co-dependent in preventing osteoporosis. "Women undergoing treatment for osteoporosis today typically are taking calcium supplements in amounts of 1,000 to 1,500 mg. of calcium per day," explains study author Dr. Robert P. Heaney. "Data shows that, in addition to providing the extra calcium a patient usually needs to slow bone loss or to support treatment induced bone gain, this amount of calcium can bind up to 500 mg. of phosphorus. Although this would present no serious problem for most people, it could impact women over 60 years old who have diets that contain less than the National Academy of Sciences recommended daily allowance of 700 mg. of phosphorus. For these women, the usual calcium supplement calcium carbonate, may block most of the absorption of phosphorus. If this happens, the calcium won't do much good because bone mineral consists of both calcium and phosphorus." [*National Osteoporosis Foundation* March 9, 2002]

Vitamin B12, Bone Health and Osteoporosis

Vitamin B12, found in dairy products, meats, poultry and fish as well as in many fortified foods such as cereals, may be an important weapon in the battle against osteoporosis. New research at Tufts' Jean Mayer USDA Human Nutrition Research Center on Aging (HNRCA) has uncovered a positive association between vitamin B12 and bone health. The Tufts researchers measured bone mineral density (a gauge of bone quality) and vitamin B12 levels in more than 2500 men and women in the Framingham Osteoporosis Study. They found that both men and women with low vitamin B12 levels also averaged lower bone mineral densities than those with higher levels. The men with low vitamin B12 levels had significantly lower bone mineral density in several areas of the hip, and women low in B12 had particularly low bone density in the spine. "This is the first large scale study of its kind to show an association between low vitamin B12 and low bone mineral density in men, and it confirms other reports of this association in women," says Katherine Tucker, PhD., director of the HNRCA's Dietary Assessment and Epidemiology Research Program. "It shows that getting enough vitamin B12 from meats, poultry, fish and dairy products may be important for both men and women in maintaining strong bones." [*Tufts University Health and Nutrition Newsletter* June 2005, Volume 23 Number 4]

Vitamin A and Fracture Risk

Both low and high levels of vitamin A up a woman's risk of hip fracture, says researchers that followed 2,799 women for 22 years. The subjects were between the ages of 50 and 74 years at the study's onset. Women who had the lowest levels of vitamin A were 90% more likely to develop hip fractures than those who had average concentrations. Also, women with the highest vitamin A levels were twice as likely to endure hip fracture compared with women who had average levels. [*American Journal of Medicine* August 1, 2004; 117: 169 - 174]

Protein and Bone Mineral Density

Increasing protein intake may help the body absorb more calcium and raise bone mineral density (BMD). The study examined protein intake and bone mineral density in 342 healthy men and women, aged 65 years or older. Subjects who consumed higher amounts of protein and calcium maintained more BMD than controls who consumed limited protein and calcium. Both are deficient in the aging population and daily requirements increase with age. [*American Journal of Clinical Nutrition* April, 2002;75: 773-9]

Vitamin D

Vitamin D is an interesting and misunderstood vitamin. It also functions as a hormone. It has gone from a 'bone nutrient' to an extraordinary molecule with far - reaching effects in a variety of cells and tissues. Vitamin D comes from two sources: sunlight which converts cholesterol in the skin to cholecalciferol (D3) or from the diet. The cholecalciferol is then transferred to the liver where it is changed to calcidiol which is in turn transferred to the kidney where it is finally changed into calcitriol. This is the active form of the vitamin. Calcitriol increases calcium and phosphorus absorption in the intestine but interestingly, there are cells in our body that can make their own calcitriol, namely breast, prostate, lung, skin, lymph nodes, colon, pancreas, adrenal medulla and brain. (Note: most of these tissues have high cancer rates so vitamin D deficiency could influence cancer rates!) Research has shown that inadequate exposure to sunlight (lack of vitamin D) is associated with an increased risk of cancer mortality for several malignancies, namely those of the breast, colon, ovary, prostate, bladder, esophagus, kidney, lung, pancreas, rectum, stomach, uterus, and non-Hodgkin's lymphoma. (Grant *Cancer* 2002; 94(6): 1867-1875). Important: Many times, despite exposure of adequate sunlight, the prevalence of vitamin D deficiency is high.

Is vitamin D safe? We have been led to believe that even low doses of fat soluble vitamin D can be toxic despite lack of evidence supporting this claim. In 1999 and 2001, Dr. Vieth (*Am J Clin Nut.* 1999; 69: 842-56 and *Am J Clin Nut* 2001

Feb;73(2): 288-94) wrote a review about the unwarranted fears in the medical community of physiological doses of vitamin D. In 1999, Dr. Vieth indirectly asked the medical community to produce any evidence 10,000 units of vitamin D a day was toxic, saying, "Throughout my preparation for this review, I was amazed at the lack of evidence supporting statements about the toxicity of moderate doses of vitamin D." He added, "If there is published evidence of toxicity in adults from an intake of 250 ug. (10,000 IU/day), I have yet to find it." Our bodies will make 10,000 - 25,000 IU of vitamin D a day with full body ultraviolet light (sunshine). Current vitamin D dosage guidelines are based solely on the maintenance of bone health and do not account for the influence of vitamin D for other physiological functions. In the absence of exposure to sunlight, a minimum of 1000 IU of vitamin D3 is required to maintain a healthy concentration of 25-hydroxyvitamin D3 in the blood.

People usually do not eat foods rich in vitamin D. Fortified foods are so variable in the amounts they actually contain that one can't rely on these as the only source of vitamin D. The most common food sources are: sardines, salmon, herring, shrimp, halibut, chicken (50 - 67 IU per 3.5 oz.), oysters, non-fat and 1% milk, yogurt (100 IU/8 oz.) and cheese. The richest sources are from seafood but there is an environmental contamination problem in many of the commercial fishing waters. In order to maximize vitamin D synthesis in the skin from sunlight one would require 15 - 20 minutes of direct sunlight exposure to the face, arms and legs, three times per week. Many people cannot do this due to skin cancer concerns, medications, or lack of sunlight in the wintertime. This is usually a problem for people who live above 42 degrees latitude. Gastrointestinal inflammatory disorders reduce dietary absorption of vitamin D. Cortisol elevations or use of cortisone can deplete vitamin D levels. Ethnicities with darker skin and individuals with obesity are more at risk for vitamin D insufficiencies.

Our vitamin D status changes as we age. By age 45 - 50, the enzyme in the kidney that makes calcitriol becomes less active and, therefore, vitamin D becomes deficient, especially in the wintertime. Studies strongly suggest that the age - related decline in calcitriol synthesis in the kidneys is a major contributing factor to the development of osteoporosis in women and men older than age 50, as well as the age - related increase in the risk of the above mentioned cancers. However, studies also indicate that individuals older than age 45 can compensate for the decline in calcitriol synthesis by raising their blood levels of the less potent form: 25-hydroxy vitamin D (calcidiol). People with autoimmune conditions usually need higher doses of vitamin D due to the prevalence of genetic vitamin D receptor polymorphisms (which means they are unable to process vitamin D the same as people without this condition).

Interesting Research

A study of 150 children and adults at the University of Minnesota found that 93% of all subjects with non - specific musculoskeletal pain were vitamin D deficient. All of the African - American, East African, Hispanic and Native American subjects were vitamin D deficient. Of these, 55% were severely deficient. "These findings are remarkably different than what is taught in medical school. We would expect vitamin D deficiency in old persons or housebound persons," says chief investigator Dr. Greg Plotnikoff. "We found the worst vitamin D deficiency in young persons - especially women of childbearing age. We were stunned to find no vitamin D at all in five patients who had been told their pain was 'all in their head'. This pain is the most common kind of complaint seen by primary care doctors." Dr. Plotnikoff points out that vitamin D deficiency is also associated with osteoporosis, hypertension, diabetes, cancer and autoimmune disease such as multiple sclerosis. Deficiency is also harmful to developing fetuses and causes rickets in children. (Mayo Clinic Proceedings Dec 2003; 78; 1463-70.)

One in seven American adolescents is vitamin D deficient, according to a study in the journal *Pediatrics* (March 2009; 123: 797-803). The study employed a new definition of vitamin D deficiency recommended by a group of scientists attending the 13th Workshop Consensus for Vitamin D Nutritional Guidelines in 2007. These experts collectively proposed that the minimum acceptable serum vitamin D level be raised from 11 nanograms per milliliter (ng/ml) to at least 20 ng/ml. Using the newer criteria, the study found more than half of African-American teens are vitamin D deficient. Girls had more than twice the risk of deficiency compared with boys and overweight teens had nearly double the risk of their normal weight counterparts.

An article in the *New England Journal of Medicine* in 1992 outlined a one and one half year study of women who were given calcium and 800 units of vitamin D3 compared to women who were given neither. The results revealed that women taking 1,200 mg. of calcium and 800 units of vitamin D3 had 43% fewer hip fractures than the other women who received none of the supplements.

Vitamin D deficiency is a major factor in osteoporosis related hip fractures, says scientists in Scotland. Specifically, out of 458 patients age 60 and older with hip fractures, 97.8% had lower than normal vitamin D levels. In a quarter of all cases, levels were so low they were effectively unrecordable. [*Current Medical Research and Opinion* August 3, 2005:21(8)]

Low vitamin D levels may also trigger hypertension or high blood pressure according to a study in the journal *Hypertension* (November 2008; 52: 828-32). Those women with the lowest levels of vitamin D had 66% bolstered risk of hypertension, compared with those with the highest levels and being vitamin D deficient increased the odds of developing high blood pressure by 47%. 'Plasma 25-OH vitamin D levels are inversely and independently associated with the risk of developing hypertension,' conclude the study's authors.

Our first line product for vitamin D supplementation is an emulsified (predigested) liquid form. Bioavailability is increased when the product is emulsified. The product also provides genistein and carnosic acid to help improve vitamin D utilization and metabolism. Genistein can optimize the 1,25 hydroxy D3 synthesis and therefore promote increased utilization of vitamin D into an active form. Carnosic acid from rosemary leaf extract has demonstrated the ability to potentiate the effects of vitamin D.

Testing for Vitamin D

There are two blood tests that should be done to monitor vitamin D status, although usually only one of the tests is done by most doctors. 25-OH vitamin D and 1,25-OH vitamin D should be done. The 1, 25-OH levels need to be done due to those genetic vitamin D receptor polymorphisms referred to earlier. These people may become vitamin D toxic even though 25-OH is normal. This is a very important point. These people will need to be supplemented differently.

Zinc

The human body contains one to two grams of zinc and about 90% is found in muscle, bone, skin and hair, while blood contains less than 1%. Zinc plays an important role in connective tissue metabolism, acting as a cofactor for several enzymes, such as alkaline phosphatase (necessary for bone mineralization), and collagenase (essential for the development of the collagenous structure of bone). Zinc deficiency results in impaired DNA synthesis and protein metabolism, which lead to negative effects on bone formation (and impaired healing). The role of zinc in bone formation is well documented in animal models, and low serum levels of zinc and excessive urinary excretion are related to osteoporosis in humans. Zinc concentration in bone is greatly reduced with zinc deficiency. Animal studies have demonstrated a beneficial effect of zinc supplementation on vertebral and femoral bone mass during strenuous treadmill exercise.

Calcium

Most people are familiar with the relationship between calcium and osteoporosis. Calcium has many physiological functions in the body, most notably:

- Bone and tooth formation
- Blood clotting
- Nerve transmission
- Skeletal muscle contraction and relaxation
- Enzyme regulation

How much do we really need? It depends on many factors such as the form of calcium and the person's unique requirements, but the National Institutes of Health has outlined some general recommendations:

Group	Optimal Daily Intake (mg.)
Infants	
Birth - 6 months	400
6 months - 1 year	800

Children

1 - 5 years	800
6 -10 years	800 - 1,000

Adolescents and Young Adults

11 - 24 years	1,200 - 1,500

Men

25 - 65 years	1,000
Over 65 years	1,500

Women

25 - 50 years	1,000

Over 50 years (postmenopausal)

On estrogen	1,000
Not on estrogen	1,500
Over 65	1,500

Pregnant or nursing	1,200 - 1,500

This is where the bioavailabity concept becomes important. This all has to do with the form of calcium and the condition of the person's gastrointestinal system which will be explained in a later chapter.

The following chart demonstrates that women's and girl's daily calcium consumption hasn't changed all that much according to USDA surveys. (Values are for daily calcium consumption in mg.)

Age Range	1988 USDA Survey	1996 USDA Survey
12 - 19	781	739
20 - 29	651	678
30 - 49	587	651
50 - 69	575	608

Do calcium supplements really help? Based on the results of more than 20 randomized trials of calcium versus placebo supplementation, calcium treatment has a small, but significantly beneficial effect on bone mineral density.

Supplemental calcium has been shown to decrease not only bone loss in post menopausal women, but also the risk of vertebral fracture, up to 45%, in women who had already suffered a vertebral fracture. Furthermore, in a large trial of 3,000 post menopausal women randomized to receive placebo or calcium and vitamin D found that by year three of the study, the probability of non-vertebral fracture and hip fracture had been reduced by 24% and 29% respectively. [*The Physician and Sports Medicine* Vol. 28; No. 2 Feb. 2000]

Remember, we should be getting the majority of our calcium from food sources. The following chart outlines some top food sources of calcium:

Food	Calcium (mg.)
Almonds (3.5 oz.)	266
Bok Choy (1 cup cooked)	230
Collard greens (1 cup cooked)	350
Mackerel (3 oz. canned w/ bones)	260
Milk (1 cup)	
Skim	302
2 percent	297
Whole	291
Rice milk (1 cup fortified)	240
Salmon (3 oz. canned)	200
Sardines (3 oz. canned w/ bones)	340
Swiss cheese (1 oz.)	250
Yogurt, plain, lowfat (1 cup)	415

| Fortified orange juice | About the same as milk |

Certain foods (butter, eggs, fatty fish) enhance calcium absorption. This is one reason why certain fats are essential in the diet.

Chapter 3

How Can Osteoporosis Be Properly Evaluated?

We have seen in the previous chapter that osteoporosis is a condition with multiple factors involved, not just calcium and vitamin D. This process is usually secondary to other issues the body is trying to contend with, so it would stand to reason that evaluation is not as simple as just doing a bone density test. The standard medical approach to determine bone mineral density is to use dual energy x-ray absorptiometry or DEXA testing. DEXA is the most common clinical test used today to measure bone density. Some advantages include:

- No radioactive isotope is used and it can measure every area of the skeleton.
- Very fast (a hip study is typically 2 - 4 minutes) and accurate with very low radiation exposure (a spine and hip study is only 1/30th the radiation of a chest x-ray).
- Precise - changes in bone density as small as 1% to 4% per year can be detected.

There are two different ways of reporting bone density scores. The first is what is termed a 'T- score'. A T- score compares your bone density to a 'young normal' healthy 30 year old adult with peak bone density. The second is termed a 'Z-score'. The Z- score compares your bone density to what is normal in someone similar in age and body size. Healthcare providers usually do not use Z-scores to diagnose osteoporosis in postmenopausal women and men age 50 and older. Decreased bone mineral density is common in older adults, therefore, Z-scores can be misleading. An older person might have a normal Z-score but still be at high risk for a fracture. Most experts recommend using Z-scores rather than T-scores for younger men, premenopausal women and children. However, T-scores are often used for perimenopausal women. A Z-score above -2.0 is normal according to the International Society for Clinical Densitometry (ISCD). *A diagnosis of osteoporosis in younger men, premenopausal women and children should not be based on a BMD test result alone.* The National Osteoporosis Foundation does not recommend routine BMD testing in children, adolescents, healthy young men or premenopausal women.

Bone densitometry measures are reported as follows.

Normal bone: T-score better than -1

Osteopenia: T-score between -1 and -2.5

Osteoporosis: T-score less than -2.5

The International Society for Clinical Densitometry recommends bone mineral density testing for the following populations:

- Women aged 65 or older
- Postmenopausal women under age 65 with risk factors
- Men aged 70 or older

- Adults with a fragility fracture
- Adults with a disease or condition associated with low bone mass or bone loss
- Adults taking medications associated with low bone mass or bone loss
- Anyone being considered for pharmacologic therapy
- Anyone being treated, to monitor the effect
- Anyone not receiving therapy in whom evidence of bone loss would lead to treatment

Scans are usually repeated every 2 to 4 years or 1 to 2 years for a specific reason.

A new method for calculating fracture risk to make decisions regarding treatment in people 40 and older is called absolute fracture risk. This is a web based tool that takes the T-score and combines other certain risk factors to predict fracture risk more accurately. This risk is basically used to determine when to start drug treatment.

There are other methods of measuring bone density such as pDXA (peripheral dual energy x-ray absorptiometry), QUS (quantitative ultrasound), QCT (quantitative computerized tomography), and pQCT (peripheral quantitative computerized tomography). QUS uses sound waves to measure bone density and all the other methods use radiation (a relatively small amount). These other methods are more for screening and the results are not quite equivalent to the central DEXA machine.

Plain film x-rays cannot be used to measure accurately bone mineral density due to the fact that 25% to 40% of density must be lost before it can be picked up on the x-ray. By the time the patient exhibits this finding they will have already lost a huge amount of bone density and the disease will be well advanced.

An interesting point is brought up by John Abramson in his book *Overdosed America.* He states that it may be hard to believe, but there has never been a randomized controlled study done to determine whether there is a benefit to screening women for osteoporosis with bone mineral density tests. There is simply no gold standard evidence showing that ordering all these tests and prescribing all those drugs is leading to better health for women.

Are there better clinical tests to use in the office? Yes. There are urine tests to determine how much bone loss is occurring at the moment. The problem with the DEXA test is that you cannot tell how much bone you are losing at the moment, it only tells you the amount you have lost up to the present. You cannot also repeat the test easily to follow treatment as insurance carriers only pay for a DEXA every one to two years.

The first test is the Osteomark® NTx urine test which is an enzyme-linked immunosorbant assay (EIA) for the measurement of cross-linked N-telopeptides of type I collagen (NTx) as an indicator of human bone resorption. What does this mean? Remember that bone is constantly being remodeled by bone resorbing cells (osteoclasts) and bone building cells (osteoblasts) and if this balance is disrupted bone structure will suffer. We can measure breakdown products in the urine and if there are too many then we know bone is being broken down faster than it is being formed and osteoporosis will eventually develop. Approximately 90% of the organic matrix of bone tissue is type I collagen which forms the basic fabric and tensile strength of this tissue. The discovery that urinary cross-linked N-telopeptides of type I collagen (NTx) provides a specific biochemical marker to quantify bone resorption and gives health practitioners a reliable and relatively inexpensive way to track treatment. Clinical research has demonstrated that elevated bone resorption is the primary cause of age related bone loss which leads to osteoporosis.

The second urine test is the DPD or D-pyridinium (Pyrilinks - D) test. This is a test for deoxypyridinoline crosslinks, which is a specific bone breakdown product. Once the breakdown products pyridinoline and deoxypyridinoline are released into the blood, they are not re-used for bone formation and neither is metabolized in the liver. They can be measured intact in the urine. Pyridinoline is a collagen degradation product derived from several tissues in addition to bone. Deoxypyridinoline is almost exclusively specific to bone tissue. This test only measures free deoxypyridinoline.

What Testing Should Be Done To Evaluate For Causes of Osteoporosis?

When functional medicine is practiced, we must look for the underlying metabolic problems that will give rise to osteoporosis and other chronic conditions, therefore, laboratory assessment will be different than just your normal bloodwork you get with your annual physical. A functional medicine assessment is much more detailed since we are interested in the relationship between symptoms, bloodwork and neurological findings, not the least number of tests we can run to keep an insurance carrier happy.

What is the basic testing we start with? The first test is a complete blood count (CBC) with differential which will tell you if you have an anemia and will also tell you if any of the different types of white blood cells are elevated (as in an infection) or decreased (as in a chronic immune challenge).

Next is a complete metabolic panel consisting of : Glucose and hemoglobin A1c, uric acid, BUN, creatinine, sodium, potassium, chloride, CO_2, calcium, phosphorus, magnesium, total protein, albumin, globulin, Albumin/Globulin ratio, total bilirubin, alkaline phosphatase, lactate dehydrogenase (LDH), SGOT, SGPT, GGT, iron, TIBC, ferritin, cholesterol, triglycerides, HDL cholesterol, LDL cholesterol, VLDL cholesterol, CRP, homocysteine, thyroid stimulating hormone (TSH), T4, T3 uptake, FTI, T3, 25-OH vitamin D, and 1,25-OH vitamin D.

A word on cholesterol: Cholesterol has been demonized by the medical community as a bad thing to have too much of. The reality is we cannot live without cholesterol. It is in every cell membrane of our body and makes up the majority of the weight of the brain along with DHA. It is a carrier for antioxidants so if we have too little cholesterol we lose much of the protection from free radical damage offered by antioxidants. This is evident from a study that reported that antibiotics and cholesterol lowering drugs may irreversibly damage the lens of the eye and cause cataracts. (*Journal of Lipid Research* - November 2002; 110: e53) We also see an increase in cancer rates, depression and suicide in patients who have low cholesterol. (*Journal of the American College of Cardiology* 2007) This is also why we see an increase in polyneuropathy in patients on long term statin therapy. Subjects who took statins were 3.7 times more likely to suffer from idiopathic polyneuropathy, compared with those who did not use statins. This risk jumped to 14.4 times among those with 'definite' polyneuropathy. Those who took statins for two years or more had the greatest risk of nerve damage. (*Neurology* - May 14, 2002; 58: 1333-7) There is a question whether statin therapy works at all. A study in the *Archives of Internal Medicine* (2010; 170(12): 1024-1031) asked if taking statins actually saved lives. For this study they used people without a history of heart disease but who were still considered to be at high or intermediate risk for heart disease. After reviewing the data from 65,229 people they found that there was no proof that these drugs saved any lives. The conclusion from the study states: "this literature based meta-analysis did not find evidence for the benefit of statin therapy on all cause mortality in a high risk primary prevention set-up." In addition, an article from the *British Medical Journal* (2010;340:c2197) links statin drugs to cataracts, liver dysfunction, myopathy (intense muscle pain) and kidney failure.

Cholesterol is also a non-specific marker for inflammation and can be raised in many conditions such as stress, infections, hypothyroidism and from too much sugar. There was a study done using the data from the National Health and Nutrition Examination Survey (NHANES) from 1999-2006. Researchers Jean A. Welsh, MPH, RN et al. of Emory University looked at the data and found with increased consumption of added sugar, average levels of HDL cholesterol were lower (the cholesterol that transports lipoprotein to the liver for disposal) and levels of triglycerides were increased. (Published in *Journal of the American Medical Association* April 21, 2010; abstract at jama.ama-assn.org/cgi/content/full/303/15/1490)

Americans get nearly 16% of total calories from sugars added to foods from manufacturing. In 1977-78 it was 10.6% of total calories. Today daily consumption averages 90 grams of added sugar, the equivalent of 21.4 teaspoons.

For further information on this topic I recommend the following books: *The Cholesterol Myths: Exposing the Fallacy That Saturated Fat and Cholesterol Cause Heart Disease* by Uffe Ravnskov, MD, PhD, *Fats That Heal Fats That Kill* by Udo Erasmus, and *Heart Disease: What Your Doctor Won't Tell You* by Dr. Rodger Murphree.

If a sudden drop or a very low level of cholesterol is detected on lab work, this is one of several 'Ominous signs'. The other indicators are : albumin below 4.0, A/G ratio below 1.0, calcium/albumin ratio above 2.7, lymphocytes below 20, absolute lymphocytes (lymphocytes divided by WBC) below 1,500, and platelets below 150 or above 450. If three or more of these labs are present then further evaluation is a must. Cholesterol is also the building block for a number of different important substances the body needs to produce as outlined in the following diagram:

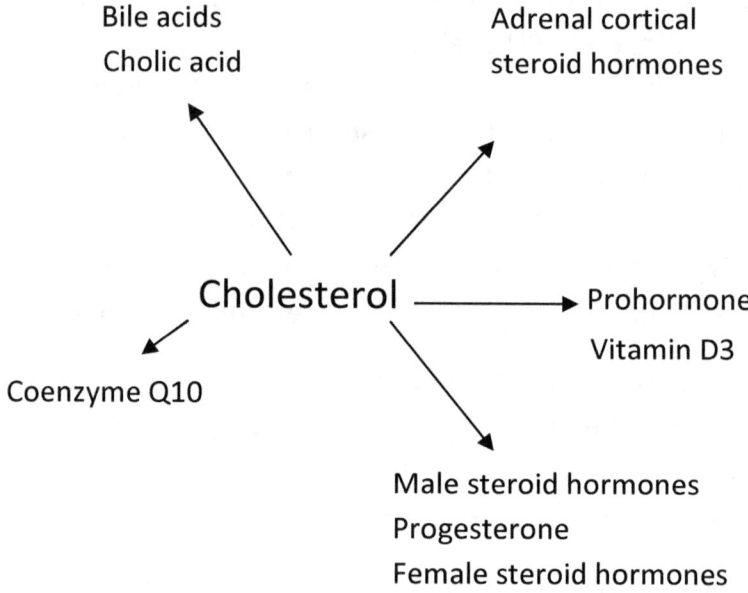

Bile acids
Cholic acid

Adrenal cortical
steroid hormones

Cholesterol ⟶ Prohormone
Vitamin D3

Coenzyme Q10

Male steroid hormones
Progesterone
Female steroid hormones

Note: When evaluating lab results, I use what are termed functional lab values rather than the ranges given by the lab itself. Functional values are more narrow than lab values and one can pick up pathological patterns far sooner than relying on the very wide laboratory values provided on the report.

An adrenal stress index should also be performed. This is a method to test the integrity of the adrenal glands (small glands which sit on top of the kidney) which are responsible for your stress response, hormone production including adrenaline/noradrenaline, blood sugar maintenance and cortisol production. And why is cortisol important?

EFFECTS OF CORTISOL

Cortisol is a hormone produced by the adrenal gland in response to stress. It follows a circadian rhythm throughout the day which is linked to patterns associated with sleeping at night and being awake during the day. Cortisol levels are typically highest in the morning and tapers down throughout the day to their lowest levels at midnight. Cortisol is ultimately controlled by the hypothalamus of the brain which is charged with maintaining homeostasis (metabolic balance) and orchestrating our responses to stress. The following is a list of the impact of cortisol on different systems of the body:

Cortisol and the Immune System

- Normally, cortisol release can happen in seconds after a stress, but if the stress is great enough the negative feedback loop is interrupted and we get too high of a cortisol response
- The number of white blood cells also fluctuates inversely with cortisol – ie. ↑cortisol = ↓white blood cells (WBCs)
- Cortisol redistributes WBCs out of the bloodstream, therefore, it affects WBC migration patterns
- Cortisol can impair the function of WBCs by inhibiting WBCs from producing pro-inflammatory cytokines – This is why cortisol is the body's own in house anti-inflammatory
- Cortisol can actually kill WBCs – cell apoptosis

- On the other hand, too little cortisol impairs the body's ability to constrain inflammation
- Dysfunctional cortisol levels are more specific for passive stresses such as depression, loss of control, helplessness rather than exercise or active stresses

Cortisol and Blood Sugar

- Elevated cortisol causes increased insulin resistance, therefore, more insulin (pro-inflammatory) is released by the pancreas
- Decreased cortisol causes hypoglycemia because it can't influence the manufacture glucose from other tissues (gluconeogenesis) or the breaking apart of stored glucose (glycolysis)

Cortisol and Thyroid Function

- Elevated cortisol has a suppressive effect on the enzyme that converts T4 (inactive thyroid hormone) to T3 (active thyroid hormone) = less active thyroid hormone

Cortisol and the Intestines

- Elevated cortisol suppresses Secretory IgA (an antibody involved in the first line of defense against invaders of mucous membranes) which delays regeneration of cells lining the intestine and promotes a pro-inflammatory environment
- Elevated cortisol contributes to dysbiosis (increase in pathogenic bacteria in the gut) and leaky gut

(increased permeability due to thinning of the GI lining) →The GI tract becomes more susceptible to parasites and other pathogenic organisms

Cortisol and Bone Density

- Elevated cortisol has a negative impact on bone metabolism due to calcium malabsorbtion

Cortisol and Insomnia

- Depressed cortisol levels leads to the inability to stay asleep due to the lack of blood sugar able to be created from gluconeogenesis and glycolysis
- If no cortisol is available for blood sugar regulation the body will use epinephrine and norepinephrine (glucocorticoids) which are excitatory hormones →wake you up
- Elevated cortisol →Hard time getting to sleep

Cortisol and the Brain

- Dysregulation of the hypothalamic/pituitary/adrenal axis (HPA axis) has been related to neurodegenerative diseases such as multiple sclerosis and lower DHEA has been linked to Alzheimer's
- Elevated cortisol has been shown to cause hippocampal cell destruction (the part of the brain associated with memory)
- Dysfunctional HPA axis can also cause an increase in pro-inflammatory cytokines leading to inflammatory damage in tissues (cardiovascular disease)→Can also

lead to an increase in blood pressure due to elevations in catacholamines

Cortisol and Metabolism

- Elevated cortisol induces insulin resistance which has been shown to lead to leptin resistance (leptin is a hormone that tells the brain to stop eating)→increased potential for obesity
- With elevated cortisol lowering the production of active thyroid hormone→slows down metabolism and fat burning
- Also, hypothyroidism shuts down the receptor sites that respond to lipase, an enzyme that metabolizes fats

Signs and Symptoms of Adrenal Stress Syndrome

Cortisol Imbalance Signs and Symptoms

- Fatigue (most common symptom)
- Headaches with physical or mental stress
- Weak immune system
- Allergies
- Slow starter in the morning
- Gastric ulcer
- Afternoon headache
- Fullness or bloated feeling

- Crave sweets, caffeine, cigarettes
- Blurred vision, unstable behavior
- Get shaky or lightheaded if meals are missed or delayed (reactive hypoglycemia)
- Irritable before meals (reactive hypoglycemia)
- Eating relieves fatigue (reactive hypoglycemia)
- Cannot stay asleep (adrenal hypofunction)
- Cannot fall asleep (adrenal hyperfunction)

An interesting finding from the American Psychosomatic Society's 67th annual meeting in Chicago (March 8, 2009) was that stress is a factor in healing of wounds. Researchers found that healing in one type of tissue may possibly worsen healing in a different type of tissue. Previous studies showed that stress is associated with reduced inflammation in skin wounds, but the effect appears to be reversed in the mucosal tissue of the palate (GI system). This may make sense from the suppression of secretory IgA (an antibody) in the GI tract by high cortisol which leads to decreased regeneration of mucosal cells and a pro-inflammatory state.

Hormone panels can also be run if indicated. We are determining if the patient has elevated or decreased DHEA, testosterone, estrogen and progesterone levels. The most effective way to test hormones is by saliva. The reason is that saliva hormone levels accurately represent the amount of hormone delivered to receptors in the body, unlike serum which represents hormone levels that may or may not be delivered to the receptors.

The majority of hormones in the blood exist in one of two forms: free (5%) or protein bound (95%). While 95% of the hormones in the body are protein bound, it is only the 5% free hormones that are biologically active. Saliva measures the free bioavailable hormone levels in the body, while serum measures only the protein bound non-bioavailable hormone levels. Also, saliva testing is much less invasive and can be done on multiple days or multiple times a day without having to do a needle stick each time.

Sensitivity testing to major food proteins should also be performed. Extensive research indicates that at least 50% of the American population develop reactions of the immune system to common dietary proteins. The most accurate test for this is a stool test for the antibodies to these proteins. The immunologic reaction to antigens begins and occurs within the intestinal tract, with antibodies passing unabsorbed, through the entire tract. It would therefore be expected that properly designed stool tests would detect antibodies much more frequently than do traditional blood tests. The lab that performs this testing also does genetic testing to see if you carry the genes for gluten reactivity called HLA - DQ genes. Once these genes are turned on they cannot be turned off. This is why if one carries the genes, gluten should be avoided for life.

Why is this a big deal? If you have an immune reaction to a certain food protein such as gluten, this inflames the lining of the intestines and will eventually lead to the leaking of the intestinal wall. This will allow the immune system to react to other food proteins such as casein or milk proteins, soy, eggs or yeast. When the immune system makes antibodies to gluten it also can make antibodies to your thyroid gland since gluten molecules and your thyroid gland look almost identical immunologically. However, this immune system attack doesn't stop at the thyroid gland. It will lead to the production of other antibodies against the cells of the stomach that produce intrinsic factor (which leads to pernicious anemia and B12 deficiency), the pancreas which leads to blood sugar control issues and the cerebellum of the brain which can lead to neurologic consequences such as balance and coordination issues. So you can see that gluten reactivity is a very serious issue especially when it will lead to malabsorption in the intestine which then will lead to osteoporosis. The point to remember is that *you can have an immune reaction to gluten and other proteins without having gastrointestinal symptoms.*

Gluten is the main protein found in wheat and other cereal grains. It is a type of prolamin, a class of simple proteins. However, not all prolamins are involved in gluten intolerance. Gluten makes dough elastic. It is a glycoprotein, which is a carbohydrate containing protein.

Glutens are divided into two broad categories: gliadins and glutenins. These two proteins are resistant to digestion by stomach acid and pancreatic enzymes. Therefore, the digestive process does not break them down into smaller components that can be more easily managed. This may be a primary factor in gluten intolerance.

Both gliadins and glutenins appear to be involved in gluten intolerance. Gliadins are rich in glutamine and proline, two amino acids. One of the glutamine rich gliadins that is particularly problematic has 33 amino acids which is a fairly large protein.

Gluten is found in:

- Wheat
- Spelt
- Rye
- Barley
- Kamut
- Durum
- Triticale
- Einkorn
- Semolina
- Bulgur
- Wheat germ
- Couscous
- Farina
- Emmer
- Matzoh
- Graham

The following grains do not contain gluten:

- Amaranth
- Buckwheat
- Corn
- Millet
- Oats
- Rice
- Sorghum
- Teff

*Note: Oats are frequently cross contaminated with wheat so only certified gluten free oats are acceptable

People with celiac disease (which is an immune response to gluten) have an elevated risk of developing osteoporosis, says an article in the *Archives of Internal Medicine*. The analysis compared 266 people with osteoporosis with 574 individuals without the bone robbing disease. The subjects were also tested for celiac disease, a disorder that frequently remains undetected. Individuals with the condition who continue to eat wheat, rye and barley have a heightened risk of intestinal cancer. Results showed biopsy proven celiac disease in 3.4% of those with osteoporosis, compared with only 0.2% among those without. A direct correlation was evident between the severity of gluten intolerance and the extent of osteoporosis. "The prevalence of celiac disease in osteoporosis patients is high enough to justify a recommendation for serologic screening of all patients with osteoporosis for celiac disease," stress the study's authors. (*Archives of Internal Medicine* January 28, 2005; 165: 393-399)

The only way to test the immune system directly is to do laboratory immune panels. These panels are not part of the normal laboratory workup and most insurance companies will not pay for these as they term the tests 'experimental'. However, we can obtain critical information that cannot be detected any other way by running what is called a T and B cell panel and cytokines. This will determine if your immune system is trying to kill something (what we term an active antigen) or if there is an immune system dysregulation (such as vitamin D deficiency, blood sugar issue etc.). On the other hand, cytokines are the chemical messengers that white blood cells use to talk to each other. We divide the immune system into what is termed TH1 and TH2. Normally these two sides of the immune system should be in balance but if certain cytokines are elevated then we call this either a TH1 dominance or a TH2 dominance depending on which cytokines are elevated. This will determine if you need to stimulate one side of the immune system to balance it.

As it turns out, any condition that increases inflammation will lead to osteoporosis. Elevated interleukin-6 in the first 10 years of menopause is a predictor of bone loss in women which suggests that pre-existing systemic inflammation increases the risk of bone loss. (*Journal of Endocrinology and Metabolism* 2001; 86(5): 2032-2042)   Interleukin-1, interleukin-6 and tumor necrosis factor alpha are very powerful stimulators of bone resorption. (*Journal of Bone Mineral Research* 1996; 11(8): 1043-1051)

An intestinal microbial test may need to be ordered. The most accurate test for this is a polymerase chain reaction (PCR) DNA test. The microbial population is measured using PCR amplification of the genetic material of each organism, allowing for sensitive detection as well as the ability to detect and identify organisms that cannot be cultured or are extremely difficult to grow under laboratory conditions. This DNA amplification tests for the genetic material of pathogenic bacteria, yeast, fungi and parasites. Many times, gut infections can be the active antigens that the immune system is reacting to. This can lead to a low grade inflammatory reaction that never calms down if the immune system cannot completely eradicate the offending organism.

Helicobacter pylori is an extremely common infection in the stomach. It is a bacterium that colonizes the gastric mucosa of more than half of the human population worldwide. A high incidence of positive antibodies has been reported in different neurological and ophthalmological disorders including cerebrovascular diseases/stroke, mild cognitive impairment, Alzheimer's disease, Parkinson's disease, seizure disorders, migraine, multiple sclerosis, peripheral neuropathies, Guillain-Barre syndrome, and glaucoma. (*The Internet Journal of Neurology* 2008: Vol 9 No. 2) H. pylori does its damage by a number of mechanisms.

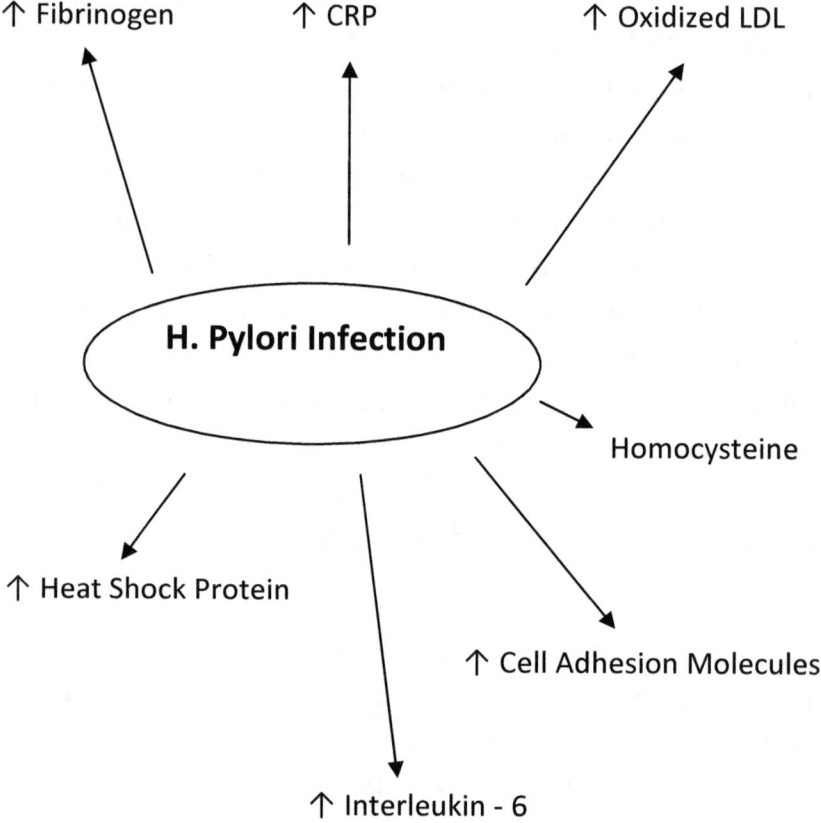

The following references illustrate the seriousness of H. pylori infections:

H. pylori promotes atherosclerosis through the generation of persistent low - grade inflammatory stimulus and is evident by the increased production of C-reactive protein. (*British Medical Journal* 1996; 27:1061-1065)

Chronic infections with H. pylori promote the production of pro-inflammatory cytokines as well as cellular adhesion molecules involved in the attachment of monocytes to the endothelial wall and promote atherogenesis. (*Circulation* 1998; 97: 1671-1674)

Cross - sectional and retrospective studies have linked H. pylori with cardiovascular disease development. (*Circulation* 1998; 97: 1675-1679)

Treatment of H. pylori and Chlamydia pneumonia infections decreases fibrinogen plasma levels in patients with ischemic heart disease. (*Circulation* 1999; 99: 155-59)

H. pylori infection causes persistent platelet activation *in vivo* through enhanced lipid peroxidation. (*Artiosclerosis, Thrombosis, and Vascular Biology* 2005; 25: 246)

If the laboratory markers for hypochlorhidria (not producing enough stomach acid) which include elevated monocytes, increased or decreased BUN, increased or decreased protein and increased or decreased globulin, a urea breath test should be performed to rule out H. pylori infection. If the test is positive, the infection should be treated along with all members of the family including the pets.

Remember from the previous chapter the consequences of decreased stomach acid on mineral absorption and bone health.

Chapter 4

What Can I Do About It?

The greatest discovery of my generation is that human beings can alter their lives by altering their attitudes of mind.

William James

The medical establishment has a straightforward approach to osteoporosis: Take calcium (usually in the form of Tums™), some vitamin D and get a bone density test every two years. If that doesn't work, then normally a bisphosphonate drug will be prescribed. Hopefully, you can see that this approach will not work from reading the previous chapters. Drug therapy for osteoporosis has a less than optimal result.

Medical Treatments

Fosamax® and Actonel® are two of the most thoroughly studied medications currently available. They work by attaching themselves to calcium in bone and inhibit osteoclast activity (cells that break down or resorb bone).

Here is the downside. These drugs must be taken on an empty stomach with a glass of water at least 30 minutes before breakfast due to poor absorption. The patient must also remain upright so the medications will not get into the esophagus as they can cause severe irritation or ulcers in some cases. The drugs are not recommended for patients with kidney failure or existing serious gastrointestinal problems.

In 1995, Fosamax® was the first of a new generation of drugs approved by the FDA for the treatment of osteoporosis. In a study in 1998 women who took Fosamax® for four years were 56% less likely to suffer a hip fracture than women in the control group. This sounds very good, but how many hip fractures were really prevented? With no drug therapy, women with osteoporosis had a 95% chance of making it through each year without a hip fracture - pretty good odds. With drug therapy, their odds improved to 99.8%. In other words, taking the drugs decreased their risk of hip fracture from 0.5% per year to 0.2% per year. This tiny decrease in absolute risk translates into the study's reported 56% reduction in relative risk. The bottom line is that 81 women with osteoporosis would have to take Fosamax® for 4.2 years, at a cost of more than $300,000, to prevent one hip fracture.

A study published in the *NEJM* in 2001 showed that even women with severe osteoporosis derived only a small benefit from these drugs. Moreover, the drug appeared to have no beneficial effect on their overall health. There was no difference in the number of serious illnesses (causing death or hospitalization), including fractures, that occurred in the women who took Actonel® compared with those that took the placebo. The same result was found in younger women. (*New England Journal of* Medicine 2001;344(5): 333-340)

A study done in the Netherlands put these lackluster results into perspective. It turns out that bone mineral density tests identify only a small part of the risk of hip fracture. The study found that for women between the ages of 60 to 80, only one sixth of their risk of fracturing a hip is identified by BMD testing. Other factors were just as important as the T-score: increased fragility, muscle weakness, the side effects of other drugs, declining vision, and cigarette smoking. As a result of the WHO study group's definition of osteoporosis, however, women and their doctors mistakenly latch on to the results of BMD testing as the sole or primary predictor of fracture risk. Routine BMD testing may not be the best way to help women prevent hip fractures, but it is an excellent way to sell more drugs. (*British Medical Journal* 1997; 315: 221-225)

In his book *Overdosed America,* John Abramson addressed the issue of using drugs to prevent osteoporosis. Fosamax® and Actonel® were approved by the FDA to treat women with osteopenia based on studies that showed that they significantly increase the bone density of these women. It is important to remember, however, that bone density is only a surrogate end point; the real reason for taking these drugs is to reduce fractures, and hip fractures in particular. The study of Fosamax® published in *Journal of the American Medical Association* in 1998 also included women with osteopenia. The results show that the risk of hip fractures actually *went up 84%* with Fosamax® treatment. (This did not reach statistical significance) The risk of wrist fractures increased by about 50%. (That figure may be statistically significant but it can't be determined from the data as presented in the article.)

Evista® was in a new class of drugs called selective estrogen receptor modulators or SERMs. These drugs are designed to protect bones the same way natural estrogen does, but without the risk of hormone therapy. Sounds great, but research shows that in women with osteoporosis, Evista® reduces only vertebral fractures, not fractures of the hip or wrist. Advertising for the manufacturer Eli Lilly misleadingly suggested that Evista did just that. A letter from the FDA in September 2000 requested that Eli Lilly 'immediately discontinue the broadcast of this violative statement' along with other marketing material that contained 'the same or similar violative claims or representations'.

How is this possible? The answer lies in our own bodies natural wisdom. Bone health requires balance between the activity of bone building cells (osteoblasts) and bone resorbing cells (osteoclasts). When bone mass starts to decline in women, the inner trabecular bone is lost more quickly than the outer cortical bone. Once the architecture of these internal struts is lost, there is no structure left onto which calcium can be added. The new bone, formed as a result of taking the osteoporosis drugs, is formed primarily on the outer part of the bone (cortical bone). This increases the score on the bone density test but does not necessarily contribute proportionately to fracture resistance.

Steroids are a significant risk factor for osteoporosis. Each year, millions of people are prescribed steroids such as prednisone, prednisolone, or other similar anti-inflammatory steroids for the treatment of autoimmune diseases such as lupus, rheumatoid arthritis, asthma, ulcerative colitis, muscle disorders, skin conditions and other diseases. When the use of these drugs exceeds a very short period of time, osteoporosis can result, because these steroids inhibit the formation of new bone. The mechanism by which this happens is very different from the mechanism whereby postmenopausal osteoporosis occurs. (Troendle G. Food and Drug Administration Medical Officer's Review of Fosamax® for the Treatment of Glucocoticoid Induced Osteoporosis, March 12, 1998)

Despite this important difference, Merck, seeking to significantly increase its market share for this drug, conducted studies to see if Fosamax®, previously approved for postmenopausal osteoporosis, could also be approved for preventing steroid induced osteoporosis. The fact that the FDA, unfortunately, approved this new use almost five years ago (year 2000) represents a triumph of Merck pressure, along with the complicity of top FDA officials, over medical evidence and against the recommendations for nonapproval by the FDA physician primarily responsible for reviewing the studies concerning the indication. (Troendle G. Food and Drug Administration Medical Officer's Review of Response to Approvable Letter for Fosamax® for the Treatment of Glucocorticoid Induced Osteoporosis, June 14, 1999: 1-22)

Fosamax® improved bone mineral density in the spine, although not as much as it does in postmenopausal osteoporosis, and reduced the occurrence of vertebral fractures. Although there was a reduction in vertebral fractures, there was a barely measureable improvement in total height (stature) of only 1.5 millimeters. Most disturbingly, it actually *increased* the total incidence of nonvertebral fractures, such as those of the foot, pelvis, ankle and hip. The FDA medical officer who opposed this approval correctly described these latter, nonvertebral fractures as more serious, more painful, and more incapacitating, than vertebral fractures. Other problems identified in the review included the fact that Fosamax® causes esophageal ulcers and irritation and, compared to placebo, increases the risk for abdominal pain. The FDA medical officer concluded, in recommending against approval, that the drug represents 'very small return for the inconvenience and the costs and risks of taking this drug.' (Troendle G. Food and Drug Administration Medical Officer's comments on Fosamax® Professional Product Labeling, June 16, 1999) The story of Fosamax® and steroid induced osteoporosis is taken from *Best Pills/Worst Pills* January 2005.

The story continues when a new bisphosphonate came out, Boniva®. *Best Pills/Worst Pills* ran an article in its October 2006 issue that warned against using Boniva® for seven years until 2010. The article read: 'The Medical Letter on Drugs and Therapeutics, known for it's independence from drug company influence, reviewed Boniva in it's August 14, 2006 issue. The publication noted the oral form of this osteoporosis drug had been shown to decrease vertebral fractures, which involves the bones that make up the spine. The drug did not show any decrease in nonvertebral fractures, such as hip fractures in postmenopausal women. There is no current evidence that the drug offers any unique therapeutic benefit over older osteoporosis drugs such as Fosamax® and Actonel®. (We saw how well these drugs worked) The FDA cleared Boniva for marketing in May 2003. Currently, both once-a-month 150 mg. tablet and a daily 2.5 mg. tablet are available on the market. In addition, the FDA approved an injectable form of the drug given once every three months, in January 2005 even though there are no studies available showing that injectable Boniva® decreases fractures in women. The FDA's approval was based on a study showing that the injectable form of the drug was "not inferior" to oral Boniva® in improving bone mineral density. The Medical Letter editors concluded their review by saying: "Boniva® is the first bisphosphonate approved for use in osteoporosis as an IV formulation given once every three months...IV Boniva® has been shown to be about as effective as oral Boniva® in increasing bone mineral density, but has not been shown to decrease fractures compared to placebo, and neither IV nor oral Boniva® has been shown to decrease nonvertebral fractures".'

Then a new side effect started to come to light. The use of bisphosphonate medications has been linked to jaw bone decay or osteonecrosis of the jaw (ONJ). Since 2001, more than 2,400 patients have reported bone death in their jaws after taking the medication to prevent or treat bone loss. Most of these patients were taking potent intravenously delivered forms of the drugs. Additionally, 120 people who were taking the drugs in the pill form have suffered from such debilitating pain that they have become bedridden or in need of walkers, crutches or wheelchairs. Osteonecrosis of the jaw occurs when the jaw does not heal after minor sugery that causes bone to be exposed. Often, the dying bone tissue must be treated with long term antibiotic therapy or be removed through surgery. Patients taking Fosamax® or other bisphosphonates should avoid having major dental work while they are on the medication due to increased risk of ONJ. Most dentists nowdays will ask if the patient are on these drugs and require the patient to go off them if major dental work is to be performed. This can be difficult as the half life of these drugs can be from ten to twelve years.

There is also evidence coming to light that suggests a possible interaction between nonsteroidal anti-inflammatory drugs (NSAIDS) and bisphosphonate drugs. Patients need to be aware that the combination can result in an increased risk of ulcers and other gastrointestinal side effects. The bisphosphonates examined included alendronate (Fosamax®), etidronate (Didronel®), ibandronate (Boniva®) and risedronate (Actonel®) combined with NSAIDs such as ibuprofen (Advil®) and naproxen (Aleve®). (*Best Pills/Worst Pills* Newsletter July 2010; Vol. 16 No. 10)

Then there were the issues with hormone replacement therapy (HRT) as outlined in the Women's Health Initiative trial of 16,000 women which was published in *Journal of the American Medical Association* July 17, 2002. Just five years into an eight and one half year study, women were told to stop taking hormone medication after tests revealed that six million American women who were currently taking the drugs might be at risk. The estrogen/progestin therapy did not decrease the risk of coronary heart disease. In fact, women in the treatment group saw their risk of heart attack increase by 29%. HRT also increased a woman's risk of invasive breast cancer by 26%; strokes by 41%; and blood clots by 100%. Lead investigators recommended that "clinicians stop prescribing this combination for long term use". Another issue with HRT was outline in *Digestive Disease Week* May 19, 2002. Investigators followed over 13,000 women for an average of three years. Findings showed that women on HRT had triple the risk of gallstones, compared with their peers who did not take HRT. The longer the women took HRT, the greater her risk.

You would think that the functional medicine model would be catching like wildfire, yet the trend is still heading in the wrong direction. Because of their drug oriented focus, America's medical practitioners are prescribing or administering 2.4 billion drugs per year. This works out to an average of almost eight prescriptions for every man, woman and child in the U.S. every year (it is now closer to twelve prescriptions). And if that statistic isn't startling enough, consider that it does not include over the counter (OTC) drugs, which, needless to say, push that number much higher. You know that there are people who are trying to live life under the influence of 16 drug prescriptions each year. There has to be, in order to keep the average at 8 prescriptions, because I don't take any. In looking at the latest Health and Human Services figures, the amount of prescriptions that can affect bones is staggering. For example:

Antidepressants - 117,813,000 scripts, antihypertensive agents - 113,078,000 scripts, and NSAIDS - 110,014,000 scripts during 2005. This paints a sad but accurate picture of the health of most medically oriented patients. (By the way, coming in at 13th on the list are 'vitamins and minerals', with 74,508,000 prescriptions per year. This works out to only one vitamin prescription for every four people in the U.S.)

A good rule to try to follow regarding medications is the Health Research Group's Seven Year Rule. You should wait seven years from the date of FDA approval to take any new drug unless it is one of those rare 'breakthrough' drugs that offers you a documented therapeutic advantage over older proven drugs. New drugs are tested in a relatively small number of people before being released, and serious adverse effects and life threatening drug interactions may not be detected until the new drug has been taken by hundreds of thousands of people. A number of new drugs have been withdrawn within their first seven years of being released. Also, warnings about serious new adverse reactions have been added to the labeling of a number of drugs, or new drug interactions have been detected, usually within the first seven years after a drug's release. (*Best Pills/Worst Pills* October 2006)

Major Medications Associated With Bone Loss or Osteoporosis:

- Thyroid hormone
- Heparin
- Anticonvulsants

- Depo - progesterone
- GnRH agonists
- Cortisone
- Prednisolone
- Lasix
- Methotrexate
- Lithium
- Isoniazide
- Aluminum antacids
- Prednisone
- Dexamethasone

A Functional Medicine Approach

As you can see, drug therapy is not an answer to osteoporosis. It is a complex physiological process that is dependent on many factors. To truly address osteoporosis, a functional approach is required to discover the underlying cause. There are four main pillars to evaluate when treating a patient. These are:

1. Anemias

2. Blood sugar/adrenal glands

3. Liver/gastrointestinal

4. Fatty acid metabolism

The reason I look at anemias and blood sugar first is that every cell in your body needs oxygen and glucose to live. Anemia deals with the oxygen carrying capacity of red blood cells and glucose is the fuel used in all cells. If either of these is compromised, then the patient cannot produce energy and they will not heal regardless of the treatment. It is also easy to forget that bone is a very metabolically active tissue as the marrow is where red blood cells and white blood cells originate. As a doctor, I need to find out what type of anemia is present. It is critical to differentiate between iron deficiency anemia, pernicious anemia or an anemia of chronic disease since the treatment will be different for each.

Blood sugar was discussed earlier and is rapidly becoming epidemic. Insulin resistance is linked to many of the same factors that lead to osteoporosis. How do we get insulin resistant?

Factors that Lead to Insulin Resistance

- Genetics - Receptor polymorphism
- Increased androgens - testosterone
- Stress via increased cortisol which down-regulates insulin receptors
- Inflammation
- Smoking
- Many dietary factors
- Obesity due to enlarged visceral adipose tissue which increase pro-inflammatory cytokines (IL-6, TNF alpha) and CRP; and decrease anti-inflammatory hormones such as adiponectin
- Inactivity

The liver is the major detoxification organ as well as a storage depot for many vitamins and minerals. If the liver is not functional then drugs, toxins and hormones cannot be cleared. The intestines are the major barrier between the inside and outside of the body (besides the skin) and the surface where nutrient absorption takes place. About 80% of our immune system is located in our gut as well as the friendly bacterial population that aids digestion and nutrient production.

Fatty acids are found in every cell membrane of the body and depending on what kind are consumed will dictate whether more pro-inflammatory or more anti-inflammatory fatty acids are incorporated into every cell membrane.

Classic Signs/Symptoms of Essential Fatty Acid Deficiency

- Tendency toward systemic inflammation
- Stiff or painful joints
- Arrhythmias
- Glucose control issues
- Neurological problems
- Vision abnormalities
- Dermatological (skin) issues
- Hormonal issues
  - ✓ Premenstrual breast pain/tenderness
  - ✓ Inadequate vaginal lubrication
  - ✓ Menstrual cramps

How much do we really need? We need to remember the 'More is not better' rule.

Grams Per Day of Total EPA/DHA

Current American Intake	0.12 grams
American Heart Association Recommendation	0.5 - 0.75 grams
Japanese	0.80 grams
Italian/Mediterranean	2.0 grams
Neo - Paleolithic Man	3.0 grams
Inuits	7 -10 grams

Too much EPA/DHA can lead to:

- Tissue oxidation/rancidification
- Immune suppression
- Increased stroke risk

Using cheap fish oils can be dangerous as well. For instance, oxidized fish oil (exposed to air) can raise triglyceride levels. Fish oils should also be third party tested to be contaminant free. The natural triglyceride form seems to be the best for absorption (almost 50% more plasma EPA/DHA using this form). There are also emulsified (or basically pre-digested form for people that have gastrointestinal issues which lead a more difficult absorption of the oils.

Another oil that should be considered is black current seed oil (an omega-6 oil). When we consume omega-6 oils found in most processed food (corn, sunflower, safflower, peanut, soybean oils), pro-inflammatory chemicals are produced. Black current seed oil is rich in gamma - linolenic acid, however, and is ultimately converted to what are called series 1 prostaglandins. These prostaglandins are beneficial as they:

- Decrease platelet stickiness (prevent heart attack/strokes
- Help the kidneys remove sodium and excess fluid from the body
- Relax blood vessels/decrease blood pressure
- Slow cholesterol production
- Decrease the inflammatory response
- Make insulin work more effectively
- Improve nerve function
- Regulate calcium metabolism
- Improve function of T-cells
- Prevent the release of arachidonic acid from cell membranes (leads to the opposite of this list)

There is one situation that trumps all four pillars: an autoimmune condition. This occurs when a patient's immune system attacks his/her own tissues. If a person is autoimmune then the immune system is the primary cause of issues with the four pillars and would need to be addressed.

Initial screening should include a Metabolic Assessment form and a Neurotransmitter Assessment form which will help pinpoint systems of the body that need to be further evaluated. These are simple questionnaires that the patient fills out rating the severity of different issues they are experiencing.

The next step is bloodwork including a complete blood count with differential (CBC with diff.), comprehensive metabolic panel, a complete thyroid panel with antibodies, and a lipid panel as discussed in the previous chapter. A urine test (Osteomark® or Pyrilinks® test) for bone loss should also be performed.

If an autoimmune condition is suspected or diagnosed, then T and B cell panels along with cytokines will need to be performed. This will reveal if there is an active antigen (something that the immune system is trying to kill such as bacteria, viruses, foods, chemicals, or metals) or if there is an immune system dysregulation such as a vitamin D deficiency, blood sugar issue etc. Vitamin D levels are important to get especially in autoimmune cases due to vitamin D's role as a T cell regulator. Food sensitivity testing should be run due to the very high rate of gluten reactivity in autoimmune patients. This immune reactivity will alter gut absorption of minerals and nutrients and thus affect bone health. Periods of hyperthyroidism as in Grave's disease will decrease bone mineral density so an accurate workup is critical. Autoimmune cases can be very complex and necessitate professional supervision.

An adrenal stress index (ASI) should be run to identify cortisol dysregulation. The issues with cortisol were discussed in the previous chapter. Cortisol has a major impact on blood sugar regulation, immune function and hormonal function, therefore, the adrenal glands must be evaluated.

Hormone panels should be performed, if indicated, to pick up any endocrine dysregulation. For women, checking the different breakdown products or metabolites of estrogen in the urine is also advisable for reduction of breast cancer risk. 2-hydroxyestrone tends to inhibit cancer growth and confers a protective effect to estrogen sensitive tissues. 16-a-hydroxyestrone actually encourages cellular growth (tumor development). A woman's (or man's) 'biochemical individuality' determines which of these metabolites predominates. Studies have shown that measuring the ratio of these two metabolites provides an important indication of risk for future development of estrogen-sensitive cancers. This is an important risk to know even if it does not directly affect bone density.

Thyroid health should always be addressed due to the impact that thyroid hormone has on our metabolism. Full thyroid panels, however, are rarely run on routine labwork, yet more than 25 million Americans suffer from thyroid dysfunction. About 7 to 8% of the general population (about 24 million people) suffer from an autoimmune thyroid condition called Hashimoto's thyroiditis. Patients with Hashimoto's have a strong correlation with pernicious anemia (intrinsic factor antibodies) which does not allow them to absorb vitamin B12 necessary for making quality bone. Essentially 100% of Hashimoto's patients are gluten intolerant and will eventually begin to produce cerebellar antibodies leading to transneural degeneration in that area of the brain. There is also a strong correlation with developing autoimmune diabetes. The reason lab work is important is that 90% of adult hypothyroidism (low thyroid hormone) is due to Hashimoto's thyroiditis, but only 10% of Hashimoto's patients show hypothyroid symptoms.

Inflammatory cytokines that were addressed earlier have a significant impact on the thyroid gland:

- Decreased thyroid stimulating hormone (TSH) production
- Decreased conversion of T4 (inactive hormone) to T3 (active hormone)
- Change in thyroid receptor site sensitivity
- Increased reverse T3 production (hormone unable to be utilized)

Thyroid hormone plays a critical role in immune cell growth and differentiation. With hypothyroidism there is a global loss of cholinergic activity (the neurotransmitter acetylcholine) which leads to a greater potential to develop cerebellar degeneration. The cerebellum located on the back underside of the brain is involved in balance and coordination of movements.

Hypothyroidism can lead to weight gain and obesity, depression, weakness, fatigue , myalgia and arthralgia (joint pain); all of these can lead to inactivity which is a significant risk factor in developing osteoporosis. Dr. William Evans, advisor to NASA and former head of the Nutrition, Physical Fitness and Rapid Rehabilitation Team of the National Space Biomedical Institute performed the Bed Rest Study which revealed that one week of complete bed rest is equivalent to one year of aging on the skeleton.

The thyroid gland and it's influence is so complex a whole book could be devoted to just this one topic. Hopefully, it is evident that proper workup is essential for a patient to achieve the results they are looking for.

One of the main keys to treating people successfully is to do adequate testing in order to be better able to diagnose and track a patient's progress. If there is not enough information then, as a doctor, I am guessing about that patient's health and I do not wish to do that.

Nutritional Considerations

Liver and digestive health is critical to not only bone health but overall health as well. The liver is an amazing organ that has many functions including carbohydrate, protein and fat metabolism, bile formation, storage of glucose as glycogen, fat soluble vitamins A, E, D, K, as well as vitamin B1, B2, B12, folic acid, fatty acids, and minerals such as iron and copper. It is also responsible for the manufacture of blood proteins such as albumin and beta globulins, inactivation of drugs and clearance of procoagulants, activated clotting factors, clearance of microorganisms by macrophages and breakdown of steroid and adrenal hormones. 80% of T4 (inactive thyroid hormone) is converted to T3 (active thyroid hormone) in the liver, large quantities of coenzyme Q10 are found in the liver, phospholipids are produced there and it is an important organ for vitamin D metabolism as well as insulin growth factors. In other words, you can't survive without your liver.

The liver operates like a series of oil filters, ridding the body of toxic substances. There are two main steps (called phase I and phase II) in liver detoxification. When substances such as drugs, pesticides, gut toxins, hormones, metabolic byproducts, histamine and stored toxins enter phase 1 in the liver they undergo biotransformation into primary metabolites and free radicals. These primary metabolites are more toxic than the original substances which can cause hepatotoxicity, damage to cell proteins, RNA, and DNA and be teratogenetic (malformations of a developing fetus). The primary metabolites then move to phase II where they undergo sulfation, amino acid conjugation, glucoronidation, glutathione conjugation and methylation to render them water soluble and are now able to be eliminated from the body via the gallbladder/bile, kidney or bowel. There are many drugs that deplete methyl donors, the most common are alcohol and birth control pills. This may produce sluggish detoxification.

If there is unbalanced detoxification such as producing phase 1 intermediates quicker than phase II can handle them, then there is an increased risk for diseases such a cancer and

Parkinson's. (*Toxicology Letter* 2004; 149(1-3): 309-34, *Rev. Environ. Health* 2002; 17(1): 51-64, *Antioxid Redox Signal* 2005; 7(5-6): 649-53). Foods that increase phase II detoxification enzymes include: cruciferous vegetables (broccoli, kale, cauliflower, Brussels sprouts, cabbage, bok choy), watercress, red beet root, Spanish black radish, garlic, and ellagic acid (in skin of red grapes). Chlorophyll also forms molecular complexes with toxins thus inactivating them preventing binding to cellular and DNA receptors. Not bad for food.

The other important organ is the gut or intestines themselves. This is the barrier between the inside and outside of the body and dictates what should pass through. The human gut also contains 10 times more bacteria than all the human cells in the entire body, about 100 trillion microorganisms. There are over 400 known bacterial species that generate intense metabolic activity and are of key importance for human health. In addition to promoting normal gastrointestinal functions and providing protection from infection, the intestinal microflora also exerts important effects on systemic metabolism and immune function. Science is just beginning to unravel the full scope of these friendly bacteria on our health.

Certain *Lactobacillus* and *Bifidobacterium* species produce vitamin B12, folate and vitamin K which are essential to bone health as we saw in the previous chapter. They are also vitally important in keeping pathogenic organisms in check, thereby, stopping the intestine from becoming an inflammatory battleground. By keeping inflammation in check, the intestine does not leak which would allow major proteins such as gluten, casein, soy, yeast and egg to pass through and create a chronic immune response that can potentially create an autoimmune condition in time.

When antibiotics are used, they not only kill the pathogenic organism but will also kill off many of the friendly bacteria in the gut. This is why probiotics (normal gut bacteria) and prebiotics (food for friendly bacteria) should be used during and after antibiotic therapy.

Scientists at the Technion - Isreal Institute of Technology have discovered that antioxidants in supplement form don't measure up to whole vegetables or fruits. In addition, they found that eating fruits and vegetables in combinations boosts their disease fighting properties because their antioxidants work together synergistically. "Whole fruits and vegetables contain a wide range of antioxidants" explains co-author, Michael Aviram. "In supplement form, however, antioxidants provide only limited benefits since they usually contain only one specific, isolated antioxidant." (*Free Radical Research* December 2002; 36:12)

Why are whole food complexes so important? There are hundreds of chemical compounds in food which work together synergistically and we really don't know which are the most important factors. Vitamins and co-factors in their natural, complex configurations are vastly different than any single, or separated or chemically manufactured, drug-like substances commonly called vitamins.

Judith DeCava has described vitamins in her book *The Real Truth About Vitamins and Antioxidants:*

> A vitamin is an extremely complex organic substance needed in very small amounts in the diet, and is essential for human life and metabolic processes: for growth, maintenance and health. The body is not capable of producing, or producing sufficient quantities of vitamins to supply its needs under normal circumstances. There are some vitamin like substances that are not considered 'essential' since the body's tissues are usually able to produce them in sufficient amounts. Sometimes they are supplied as composite parts of vitamin complexes of other nutrients. Each vitamin has its own unique functions in the body and cannot be replaced by any other substance. Vitamins, as coenzymes, perform principally as regulators of metabolic (all physical and chemical changes) processes and play important roles in energy production.
>
> Vitamins are obtained from foods and are an intregral part of a nutritive mixture or compound which is exquisitely interlaced and fused with the whole food itself. Some vitamins serve as 'provitamins' or as a precursor form; that is, they are converted into the required active substance within the body. Although considered a single substance, each vitamin is actually a 'group of chemically related compounds'. Separating (fractioning) the group or the compounds into single,

incomplete vitamin portions convert it from a physiological, biochemical, active micronutrient into a disabled, debilitated chemical of little or no value to living cells.

This is why I keep coming back to dietary changes and the concept of eating real whole foods. One cannot counter a terrible diet with a few isolated supplements and think that all is well. Food is much more complex than this and is the basis for all human healing.

A great book outlining the health benefits of whole food and eating by color (reds, oranges, yellows, greens and purple - and I'm not talking artificial color) is *The Color Code: A Revolutionary Eating Plan for Optimum Health* by James Joseph PhD, Daniel Nadeau, MD and Anne Underwood. (Hyperion Books 2002)

How are we doing with getting these nutrients? In the March 16, 2007 issue of the Center for Disease Control's *Morbidity and Mortality Weekly Report,* there was an article which reviewed consumption of fruits and vegetables within the U.S. population. In short, about 70% of adults did not eat at least two fruit and three vegetable servings per day. This eating pattern is terrible and speaks to one's future goals. Indeed, eating this way represents the 'Pursuit of disease'.

People need to appreciate that our present behavior represents the 'present time' manifestation of future goals. If adequate fruits and vegetables are not eaten, then the dietary goal becomes one of chronic disease. In reality, we should probably be eating five to ten times the recommended amount of vegetables and fruits, which would put us at about 750 - 1500 calories per day. However, most people currently do not get even 100 calories worth of fruits and vegetables per day which is a bit scary for the generations to come.

An interesting note: Tea can be good for bones. Drinking tea on a regular basis for ten or more years may have beneficial effects on bone density. Investigators asked 497 Chinese men and 540 Chinese women, 30 years and older, about their tea consumption and lifestyle factors. The study participants then had bone mineral density measurements for their total body, lumbar spine and hip. In total, 48.4% of subjects were habitual tea drinkers, with a mean duration of tea consumption of approximately 10 years. "Compared with non-habitual tea drinkers, subjects with habitual tea consumption of 6 to 10 years showed higher lumbar spine bone mineral densities, and those with consumption of more than 10 years showed the highest bone mineral densities of all measured regions," the authors reported. (*Archives of Internal Medicine* May 12, 2002; 162: 1001 -1006)

Data from a randomized, double-blind, placebo controlled, year long clinical trial suggest that supplementation with dietary genistein (54 mg./day) may be as effective as hormone replacement therapy in attenuating menopause related bone loss without causing the associated side effects. (*Nutr Rev* 2003 October; 61(10): 346-51)

Three Foods To Avoid

The first food is alcohol. I am giving a fairly detailed explanation to show how nutrition and, therefore, bone health is impacted by alcohol since it is so prevalent in our society.

Alcohols are organic compounds that arise naturally from the fermentation of carbohydrates in certain microorganisms. Most alcohols are toxic. They have the ability to dissolve the lipids out of cell membranes allowing the alcohol to penetrate rapidly into cells, destroying cell structures and killing cells. Ethanol, the type of alcohol we drink, is less toxic but still a drug (a substance that can modify one or more of the body's functions). From the moment alcohol enters the body, the tiny molecules need no digestion and are quickly absorbed. About 20% of the alcohol molecules are absorbed right through the walls of an empty stomach and can reach the brain within a minute. The stomach produces a small amount of an enzyme that breaks down alcohol (alcohol dehydrogenase) and can thus reduce the amount entering the blood. Men have more of this enzyme than women. The alcohol that leaves the stomach is then absorbed in the intestines and circulates through the bloodstream to the liver. Liver and stomach cells are the only cells that can produce alcohol dehydrogenase. The amount of alcohol that the liver can break down is limited to about ½ ounce of alcohol per hour, and the maximum amount is determined by the amount of alcohol dehydrogenase. The extra alcohol travels to all parts of the body, circulating until the liver can finally process it. Alcohol metabolism disrupts the liver. The liver prefers fatty acids for energy since it can package excess into triglycerides and ship them out to other tissues. When metabolizing alcohol, liver cells are forced to metabolize the alcohol, and fatty acids accumulate. The presence of alcohol in the liver can also alter protein metabolism. Synthesis of some proteins important in the immune system slows down, weakening the body's defences against infection. With excessive alcohol consumption, protein deficiency can develop. Alcohol calories are not utilized as carbohydrate calories. A molecule involved in energy production, known as NADH, is required for the metabolism of alcohol and is thus not available to produce energy from glucose. The energy cycle is blocked, fatty acids accumulate and hydrogen ions change the pH in the body. Alcohol is non-nutritive, displacing nutrients from the diet, and can effect every tissue's metabolism due to the loss of those nutrients. Stomach cells begin to over secrete acid and histamine. These changes make the stomach and esophagus lining vulnerable to ulcer formation. Intestinal cells fail to absorb B vitamins (thiamine, folate and vitamin B12). Most dramatic is the effect on folate. When alcohol is present, folate is removed from all sites of action and storage. The liver secretes folate into the blood and as the blood concentration rises the kidneys excrete the folate. Liver cells lose efficiency in activating vitamin D and alter their production and excretion of bile. Alcohol is also dehydrating. The water loss includes loss of important minerals such as magnesium, potassium, calcium and zinc. The latest evidence concerning possible cardiovascular benefits of alcohol seems to be that light to moderate consumption (for men 2 or less drinks and for women 1 drink per day) confers the greatest benefits without increased risk of breast cancer and prostate cancer. In most circumstances, possible benefits are far outweighed by the negatives of possible nutrient deficiencies, especially when talking about bone health.

The second food is fructose as high fructose corn syrup (HFCS). Fructose is a simple sugar that occurs naturally in fruit and honey. It has a lower glycemic index than glucose which means it is absorbed more slowly into the bloodstream. There is nothing wrong with eating fructose in fruits and moderate amounts of honey since fruits and honey contain an abundance of minerals, antioxidants, and/or fiber and other beneficial phytonutrients. Fructose by itself, however, is a major problem. In the last 25 to 30 years, in the form of high fructose corn syrup has become one of the primary sweeteners in our food supply. Look on food labels - *It is in almost everything processed we eat!* There are 60 items on the McDonald's nutrition handout and 45 of them contain HFCS. Corn syrup alone is composed mainly of glucose. HFCS is a concentrated product produced by converting much of the glucose to fructose. Food companies like it because it is less expensive but sweeter than cane sugar. (This is what allows them to 'supersize' those soft drinks for nearly the same cost as a smaller drink.) Undoubtedly, the public's major source of HFCS comes from soft drinks, but it's hard to find any sweetened food product that doesn't now contain HFCS. In the 1970's per capita consumption of HFCS was less than one pound per year; it now exceeds 60 pounds per year. Never in history have humans consumed as much fructose, and never has there been such a widespread problem with obesity. To manage weight effectively, people need to minimize their consumption of HFCS.

When one consumes carbohydrates other than fructose, the pancreas releases insulin. Insulin allows glucose to enter the cells to be used for energy. Insulin also triggers a signal to the brain that tells it that you are satisfied and full. Insulin also stimulates the production of the hormone leptin. Leptin is produced by your fat cells, which limits fat storage and helps to increase your metabolic rate to burn excess fat. Fructose does not trigger the release of insulin, therefore, it isn't moved into muscle cells for energy very well, leptin production isn't stimulated, and your metabolism doesn't increase. You also don't feel full with a large intake of fructose. These facts have lead many researchers to conclude that HFCS is one major underlying cause of the unprecedented obesity problem we are facing today.

Another troubling effect of consuming HFCS is rapid development of atherosclerosis or heart disease. In a study presented at the American Diabetes Association scientific meeting, University of California Davis researchers reported that overweight men and women who got 25% of their calories from fructose sweetened beverages developed signs of atherosclerosis in as little as *two weeks*.

If you eat any processed foods (and we all do) it's practically impossible to avoid all HFCS sweetened products. It would be wise to check food labels and avoid HFCS when possible, particularly when it is one of the main ingredients.

The last food to avoid is hydrogenated oil as trans fatty acids. To increase the marketability of cholesterol free, polyunsaturated oils, the food industry devised a method to convert liquid oils into semisolid fats. Hydrogen is 'bubbled' through the liquid oils until they became chemically saturated. Adding the extra hydrogen atoms onto the fat molecule turns an unsaturated fat into a saturated fat and allows these new products to compete with butter and lard. This is bad enough, but hydrogenation also produces some pretty strange fat molecules that aren't naturally found in the human food chain. Trans fatty acids are formed when oils are partially hydrogenated and are only useful as energy. They are not useable in cell membrane structure or immune function, unlike the natural cis - form essential fatty acids. Trans fatty acids have been shown to increase blood cholesterol levels by as much as 15% and triglyceride levels by as much as 47%. Recent research indicates that trans fatty acids are eaten in much larger amounts than saturated fats, and is now a greater risk factor for heart disease than saturated fats. *There is no safe amount of trans fats!* As of 2004, food manufacturers are required to put the amount of trans fats in their product on the nutrition labels. The fact that hydrogenated fats don't smoke or burn at higher temperatures makes them ideal to use in deep frying. They don't absorb any flavor from food, so chicken, fish, and onion rings can all be fried in the same grease. And best of all the customer can't taste any difference when the oil becomes rancid. This last little feature makes hydrogenated oils a popular ingredient for cookies and crackers that need a longer shelf life. By the time a hydrogenated fat reaches your kitchen, it doesn't even resemble the original oil that comes from the seed or nut. Estimates are that 50 - 75% of fats now consumed in the U.S. are hydrogenated.

For decades, nutritionists, physicians, and health publications have sold the public on the idea that margarine is 'heart smart' and is even served in hospitals! Margarine is a product of hydrogenation, and is far more dangerous to your health than butter. The fats it contains are not compatible with our body chemistry, and studies from as early as the 1950's have shown that these man made, hardened oils are dangerous. They have a higher melting point than our body temperatures, which allows them to circulate in the bloodstream as a solid fat rather than an oil. They contribute to heart and artery disease, arthritis, nerve disease, and cataracts. Steer clear of 'hydrogenated' foods.

Exercise and Physical Activity For Prevention of Fractures

Lack of activity destroys the good condition of every human being while movement and methodical exercise save it and preserve it.

Plato

It doesn't matter if you were once physically active in your younger years; if you're not currently engaged in a physical activity program on a regular basis, your body is not receiving the innumerable health related benefits of exercise. To show how important physical activity is, I will give you 48 reasons to exercise no matter your age.

1. Improves immune system functioning.
2. Helps you lose weight and maintain weight loss, especially body fat weight.
3. Improves survival rate from myocardial infarction.
4. Improves body posture.
5. Reduces risk of heart disease.
6. Improves the body's ability to use fat for energy during physical activity.
7. Helps the body resist upper respiratory tract infections.
8. Helps relieve the pain of tension headaches.
9. Increases maximum oxygen uptake.
10. Increases muscle strength.
11. Helps preserve lean body tissue.
12. Reduces the risk of developing high blood pressure.
13. Increases density and breaking strength of ligaments and tendons.
14. Improves coronary heart circulation.
15. Increases levels of HDL cholesterol and reduces LDL cholesterol.
16. Helps improve short-term memory.
17. Sharpens dynamic vision and controls glaucoma.

18. Reduces risk of developing type II diabetes (non insulin dependent)
19. Reduces anxiety.
20. Assists in quitting smoking.
21. Slows the rate of joint degeneration (osteoarthritis).
22. Enhances sexual desire, performance and satisfaction.
23. Helps in management of stress.
24. Improves quality of sleep.
25. Reduces the risk of developing colon cancer.
26. Reduces the risk of developing prostate cancer.
27. Reduces the risk of developing breast cancer.
28. Reduces the risk of developing a stroke.
29. Reduces susceptibility to coronary thrombosis (a clot in the artery that supplies the heart with blood).
30. Helps alleviate depression.
31. Helps alleviate low back pain.
32. Improves mental alertness and reaction time.
33. Improves physical appearance.
34. Improves self esteem.
35. Decreases resting heart rate.
36. Helps in relaxation.
37. Helps prevent and relieve the stresses that cause carpal tunnel syndrome.
38. Helps relieve constipation.
39. Protects against 'creeping obesity' (slow weight gain that occurs with age)
40. Improves blood circulation, resulting in better functioning of organs, including the brain.
41. Increases productivity at work.
42. Improves balance and coordination.

43. Helps to retard bone loss as you age, thereby reducing the risk of developing osteoporosis.
44. Improves general mood state.
45. Helps in maintaining an independent lifestyle.
46. Allows more energy and vigor to meet the demands of daily life.
47. Increases overall health awareness.
48. Improves overall quality of life.

Our brains were built for movement and our ancestors walked an estimated 12 miles per day. A lifetime of exercise can result in an astonishing elevation of cognitive abilities and performance, compared to sedentary individuals. Exercisers outperform couch potatoes in tests that measure long-term memory, reasoning, attention, problem-solving and even so-called fluid intelligence tests. These tasks test the ability to reason quickly and think abstractly.

Exercise helps our brains by providing better access for delivery of glucose and oxygen and removal of toxic waste. Brains are constantly utilizing an incredible amount of energy: even though it represents only 2% of most people's body weight, it accounts for about 20% of the body's total energy usage. When the brain is fully working, it uses more energy per unit of tissue weight than a fully exercising quadriceps leg muscle. In fact, the human brain cannot simultaneously activate more than 2% of its neurons at any one time. More than this, and the glucose supply becomes so quickly exhausted that you will faint.

Our brains need oxygen rich blood to carry away the toxic waste generated from use. How much waste is accumulated? Think about it this way. Three requirements for human life are food, drink and air but their effects on survival have very different timelines. You can live for 30 days or so without food and about a week or so without water, but the brain cannot go for more than five minutes without oxygen without risking serious and permanent damage. Toxic electrons over-accumulate because the blood can't deliver enough oxygen 'sponges', and finally rid the brain of these offenders as carbon dioxide.

When you exercise, blood flow to body tissues is increased. Exercise stimulates the blood vessels to create nitric oxide, a powerful flow regulating molecule, which helps the body make new blood vessels capable of penetrating deeper into tissues. The more exercise the better the transportation system can deliver more oxygen and remove more waste.

Exercise also works a different way. It stimulates one of the brain's most powerful growth factors, BDNF or Brain Derived Neurotrophic Factor which acts as fertilizer. This protein keeps neurons young and healthy, rendering them much more willing to connect with one another. It also encourages neurogenesis, the formation of new cells in the brain. The cells most sensitive to this are in the hippocampus, inside the very regions deeply involved in human cognition. Exercise increases the levels of usable BDNF inside those cells. The more you exercise, the more fertilizer you create.

One easy treatment for increasing bone mass in premenopausal women was explained by Dr. Joan Bassey, a physiologist from Nottingham, England. Dr. Bassey tested premenopausal women who performed a maximum of 50 heel drops, six days a week. When performed properly, each heel drop repetition was equal to the force of three times the person's body weight dropping onto the floor. Dr. Bassey found that after five months, the heel drops resulted in a 3% jump in bone mineral density in the premenopausal women. This jump was not seen in the postmenopausal group and the reason is unclear.

Research presented at the 24th annual meeting of the American Society for Bone and Mineral Research reveals that back strengthening exercises may ward off osteoporosis related spinal fractures. Members of the experimental group had ⅓ the rate of vertebral fractures, compared to controls that did not perform the exercises. In addition, bone mineral density was significantly higher in the exercising group. (*American Society for Bone and Mineral Research* September 20, 2002)

The level of exercise required to affect bone mineral density is 3 mph for 50 minutes at 5 days per week for aerobic activity. Bone mineral density is not significantly affected in the upper body with aerobic activity. Strength training is essential for maintaining bone density and balance training is essential for maintaining balance and preventing falls. This all boils down to Wolff's Law.

In a study of typical older people (ages 55 to 75), who unfortunately do not participate in regular vigorous exercise, daily activities and low intensity exercise like walking appeared to be relatively ineffective for preventing age related bone loss. (*Journal of Internal Medicine* November 2002)

Moderate walking does appear to reduce hip fracture rate. Investigators tracked 61,200 healthy postmenopausal women for twelve years. During that period, 415 suffered hip fractures. After adjusting for known risks for hip fracture, the study's authors found women cut their risk by 6% for each hour of moderate walking they engaged in a week. Those that walked at least 4 hours per week (but took part in no other exercise) showed a 41% reduced risk. In addition, standing for more than ten hours per week cut the risk of hip fracture by 28%. Subjects who stood for more than 55 hours per week enjoyed a 46% lower risk. (*Journal of the American Medical Association* November 2002; 288: 230-236)

Exercise is more influential than calcium intake in determining bone strength in young women, finds a study that tracked 80 mostly Caucasian young women for 10 years. "Although calcium intake is often cited as the most important factor for healthy bones, our study suggests that exercise is really the predominant lifestyle determinant of bone strength in young women," says lead investigator Tom Lloyd, PhD. "There was also a small positive relationship between calcium intake and bone variables, but a significant association between sports exercise score and young adult bone mass and strength. Our statistical analysis of sport - exercise in adolescence showed that exercise is responsible for between 16% and 22% of the variation in hip bone mineral density and bending strength." Dr. Lloyd points out that a female's bone mass is built between the ages of 13 and 15 and is then slowly lost in the last four decades of her life. Therefore, attaining optimal bone mass and bone strength in adolescence may offer the best protection possible against osteoporosis related bone loss in postmenopausal women and the elderly. (*Pediatrics* July 2004; 106:4)

Maintaining the mineral mass of the skeleton is important to preventing osteoporosis in an aging population. Exercise, especially weight bearing, has long been recognized as a strategy to build and maintain strong bones, and therefore, master athletes might be expected to have greater bone mineral density than inactive adults. Souminen and Rahkila studied bone mineral density, using the heel bone, in 111 male athletes who were active in the Finnish sports organizations for master athletes. The participants ranged in age from 70 to 81 years old and athletes from several sports (runners, cross-country skiers, sprinters, jumpers and weightlifters) were included. Master athletes had superior bone density (19 - 28% higher), even at advanced ages, compared to the average older male in the population. (*Med Sci Sports Exer* 1991; 23: 1227-1233) An important idea considering that by age 74, ½ of males and ⅔ of females can't lift a gallon of milk (8 pounds).

What happens when we stop exercising? Gains in bone mineral density do not appear to be preserved when the exercise is discontinued, according to the American College of Sports Medicine. Therefore, consistency is the key.

Neurological Assessment

Functional neurology is a field which is completely absent from modern medicine in the clinical setting, yet is one of the most important aspects of a patient's diagnostic workup and treatment. The brain is constantly rewiring and changing which is a process called plasticity. If you give a nerve cell what it needs to survive (fuel and activation), they can become stronger. The old adage "Use it or lose it" is true in this circumstance.

The starting point for all health is the survival of neurons or nerve cells. They require fuel in the form of glucose along with oxygen and activation which are impulses from your everyday sensory experience. This is the reason diabetes and anemia are dangerous since cells do not get adequate glucose and oxygen respectively. If this is the case, then the patient cannot produce energy to carry out all of the bodily functions necessary for growth and repair.

Different parts of the brain are responsible for different functions. Simply, the human brain has three major parts:

1. Cortex - the top of the brain where higher functions occur.
2. Cerebellum - back of the brain - involved with movement coordination and balance.

3. Brain stem - connects to spinal cord and involved with lower automatic functions such as heart rate and breathing. It can be divided into three parts: upper, middle and lower.

The cortex can be divided into right and left brain (hemispheres). They each have different properties associated with them, for example:

Right Brain	**Left Brain**
Withdrawal responses	Rote memorization
Sees the whole	Linear
Social skills	Likes routine
Reading/math comprehension	Generates positive emotions
Infers	Serial calculation
Generates negative emotions (fear, sad)	Intention, motivation
Timing, prediction	Verbal communication
Nonverbal communication	Pleasant smells
Non-pleasant smells	See familiar faces
Environmental sounds (blue, green, purple)	High frequency stimuli

Right Brain	**Left Brain**
Low frequency stimuli (red, orange, yellow)	'What' memory
'Where' memory	Approach responses
See unfamiliar faces	Impulsive, hyperactive brain

Decreased output of the cerebellum can lead to:

- Vertigo (often mistaken for inner ear problems)
- Neck and back pain
- Loss of coordination

Decreased output of the lower brainstem can lead to:

- Nausea and vomiting
- Heart arrhythmias
- Breathing problems
- Urinary tract infections
- Irritable bowel syndrome
- Constipation

Upper brainstem dysfunction can lead to:

- Chronic pain
- Light sensitivity
- Insomnia
- Restless leg syndrome
- Migraines

- Fibromyalgia
- TMJ dysfunction

One can see why increasing the 'frequency of firing' of the neuronal areas that are not working well is critical. How do we accomplish this? By using modalities such as:

- ✓ Unilateral manipulation
- ✓ Upper body ergometer
- ✓ Vibration therapy
- ✓ Warm water calorics
- ✓ Spin therapy
- ✓ Physical therapy modalities
- ✓ Interactive metronome
- ✓ Sound therapy
- ✓ Visual therapy
- ✓ Olfactory stimulation
- ✓ Eye exercises
- ✓ Spinal decompression
- ✓ Class IV laser therapy

There are many more treatment options but the bottom line is to get the proper stimulation into the proper area to functionally regulate the nervous system.

Osteopenia and osteoporosis are associated with idiopathic (origin unknown) benign positional vertigo (BPV). A study in the journal *Neurology* (March 2009; 72: 1069-76) compared 209 individuals with BPV and 202 control subjects. Bone mineral density testing revealed that BPV patients were significantly more likely to have osteopenia or osteoporosis, compared with control subjects. The study's authors theorize that a problem with calcium metabolism may be associated with BPV.

This shows that treatment needs to focus on the neurological component as well as the metabolic component.

Prevention of Fractures

Each year 32,000 older adults suffer from hip fractures attributable to drug - induced falls resulting in more than 1,500 deaths. In one study, the main categories of drugs responsible for the falls leading to hip fractures were sleeping pills and minor tranquilizers (30%), antipsychotic drugs (52%), and antidepressants (17%). All of these categories of drugs are often prescribed unnecessarily, especially in older adults. Other factors which increase the risk of falling are poor vision, dementia, neurological disorders such as stroke or Parkinson's disease, alcoholism and muscular problems.

Consider these facts:

- In an average year, 20% to 30% of people 65 years of age and older will fall.
- Of people over the age of 80, some 50% will fall at least once.
- Accidental deaths, most of which are due to falls, are the sixth leading cause of death in the elderly.

- The National Osteoporosis Foundation in Washington D.C., states that 50,000 deaths occur each year from hip fractures that result from falls.
- Falling is also listed as a contributing factor in 40% of nursing home admissions.

What can be done to prevent falls?

- ✓ Brain based therapy, correcting musculoskeletal misalignment, muscle weakness, poor coordination and lack of agility are important factors to be addressed.
- ✓ Visual problems need to be addressed; near - sightedness, far - sightedness, cataracts, macular degeneration and glaucoma. Vision is by far our most dominant sense, taking up half of our brain's resources.
- ✓ Prevention in the home; safety rails, proper shoes, non-skid mats, proper lighting and clearing obstacles to prevent tripping.
- ✓ Balance training should be done by everyone, regardless of age. This can be done using certain balance exercises on a floor (standing on one foot, using foam rollers, stability balls or a balance mat).

Conclusion

Strong Reasons make Strong Actions

William Shakespeare (1564-1616)

The human body really is amazing. Consider these facts:

- A fully formed human brain contains 100 billion neurons or nerve cells and gives off the equivalent power of a 20 watt light bulb.
- The human brain has the storage capacity of 100 trillion bits of information over the course of 70 years, equal to 500,000 sets of encyclopedias.
- Breathing one pint of air 17 times a minute, we take in 78 million gallons in an average lifespan, enough to fill the Hindenburg airship one and one half times.
- You have 45 miles of nerves in your body that send impulses as rapidly as 325 miles per hour. Your brain and your body communicate instantly.
- 8,000,000 new red blood cells are produced in the bone marrow every second.
- 2,100 gallons of blood are pumped through 62,000 miles of blood vessels in a day.
- Your heart pumps enough blood in an average lifetime to fill the fuel tanks of 56 moon rockets.
- The heart weighs less than one pound and yet beats approximately 40 million times per year.
- The lungs use about 90 gallons of pure oxygen per day.

- Because of the alveoli (tiny air sacs in the lungs), the surface area of the lungs is approximately 40-60 square miles.
- Stomach acid (hydrochloric acid) is so strong, that one drop of it on the skin will leave a painful blister, but the stomach is left unharmed.
- The stomach produces 2.5 quarts of acid per day.

Your body is a self healing entity but it needs the right raw materials to get the job done. Drugs, surgery and emergency care are like the fire department putting out fires. Functional medicine should be the construction company coming to repair and rebuild. In our modern disease care system the construction company usually doesn't show up. We all basically require the same things:

1. Aerobic activity

2. Physical (strength) activity

3. Essential fatty acids

4. Vegetables and fruits

5. Adequate protein

6. Rest

7. Good social contacts

8. Proper hydration/fluids

The prevalence in modern society of many chronic diseases such as osteoporosis is the consequence of a mismatch between modern dietary patterns and the type of diet that our cells require. Physiology is the genetic expression of one's lifestyle choices (type II diabetes, obesity, hypertension, insulin resistance, dyslipidemia, osteoporosis). These conditions can be changed given the right diagnosis, lifestyle changes and time.

Doctors William Evans and Irwin Rosenberg wrote a book that outlined the ten determinants of aging. (*Biomarkers: The 10 Determinants of Aging You Can Control* New York: Simon and Schuster 1991) All the biomarkers mentioned can be controlled and changed by lifestyle factors which give every choice we make tremendous significance. The biomarkers are:

- ✓ Muscle mass
- ✓ Strength
- ✓ Basal metabolic rate
- ✓ Body fat percentage
- ✓ Aerobic capacity
- ✓ Blood sugar tolerance
- ✓ Cholesterol/HDL tolerance
- ✓ Blood pressure
- ✓ Bone density
- ✓ Ability to regulate internal body temperature

Notice that bone density is on the list. A health practitioner addressing the issue of osteoporosis must include several items in a workup of the patient. These include:

- ✓ A thorough history and records review
- ✓ A food diary
- ✓ A metabolic assessment and neurotransmitter assessment form
- ✓ Proper labwork (CBC, chemistry panel, lipid panel, thyroid panel, sensitivity testing, adrenal stress index, hormone panel, immune panels, bone resorption urine test, GI microbial assessment, urea breath test)
- ✓ Neurological assessment
- ✓ Physical activity recommendations

Health is one of the greatest gifts we are given. Most don't think about health until it is lost. When health is absent:

- Wisdom cannot reveal itself
- Art cannot be expressed
- Wealth is useless
- We can't be there for others
- We cannot contribute our gifts and talents to the world

I hope I have impressed upon you that osteoporosis is much more complex than a lack of calcium and vitamin D. It is a condition that is secondary to other pathologies which must be managed in order for osteoporosis treatment to ever benefit the patient. It is also about prevention from infancy since this is the stage where chronic conditions begin.

I wish to thank all my past and present patients for allowing me to serve and learn from them.

Since I am a chiropractor, I thought I would end this book with a quote from the late George Sheehan about how the patient will get the optimal results if treated metabolically, neurologically and structurally.

THE HUMAN BODY IS A MARVELOUS INSTRUMENT. WHEN IN PERFECT ALIGNMENT AND BALANCE, THERE IS ALMOST NO FEAT OF ENDURANCE THE BODY CANNOT HANDLE, EVEN ON A REGULAR BASIS. HOWEVER, STRUCTURAL IMBALANCE OF EVEN MINOR DEGREES CAN RESULT IN INCAPACITATING INJURIES AND PERSISTENT DISABILITIES.

GEORGE SHEEHAN, M.D. CARDIOLOGIST

The Ambulance Down in the Valley

'Twas a dangerous cliff, as they freely confessed,
Though to walk near its crest was so pleasant,
But over its terrible edge there had slipped,
A duke and full many a peasant.

So the people said something would have to be done,
But their projects did not at all tally.
Some said, "Put a fence around the edge of the cliff,"
Some, "An ambulance down in the valley."

But the cry for the ambulance carried the day,
For it spread through the neighboring city,
A fence may be useful or not, it is true,
But each heart became moved with pity,

For those that slipped over that dangerous cliff;
And the dwellers on highway and alley,
Gave pounds and gave pence not to put up a fence,
But an ambulance down in the valley.

Then an old sage remarked, "It's a marvel to me
That people give far more attention
To repairing the results than to stopping the cause,
When they'd much better aim at prevention.

"Let us stop at its source all this hurt," cried he.
"Come, neighbors and friends, let us rally.
If the cliff we will fence, we might almost dispense
With the ambulance down in the valley."

Joseph Malens 1895

To contact the author please e-mail at:

drmiller@miller-chiro.com